Patients' Guide to

Brain Cancer

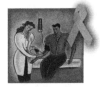

Deanna Glass-Macenka, RN, BSN, CNRN

Program Coordinator
Brain Tumor Program, Department of Neurosurgery
The Johns Hopkins Hospital
Baltimore, MD

Alessandro Olivi, MD

Professor of Neurosurgery and Oncology
Director of Neurosurgical Oncology
Vice Chairman, Department of Neurosurgery
The Johns Hopkins Hospital
Baltimore, MD

SERIES EDITORS
Lillie D. Shockney, RN, BS, MAS

University Distinguished Service Associate Professor of Breast Cancer; Administrative Director of Breast Cancer; Associate Professor, Department of Surgery; Associate Professor, Department of Obstetrics and Gynecology, Johns Hopkins School of Medicine; Associate Professor, Johns Hopkins School of Nursing

Gary R. Shapiro, MD

Chairman, Department of Oncology
Johns Hopkins Bayview Medical Center
Director, Johns Hopkins Geriatric Oncology Program
The Sidney Kimmel Comprehensive Cancer Center at Johns Hopkins, Baltimore, MD

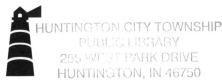

JONES & BARTLETT
L E A R N I N G

World Headquarters

Jones & Bartlett Learning
40 Tall Pine Drive
Sudbury, MA 01776
978-443-5000
info@jblearning.com
www.jblearning.com

Jones & Bartlett Learning
Canada
6339 Ormindale Way
Mississauga, Ontario L5V 1J2
Canada

Jones & Bartlett Learning
International
Barb House, Barb Mews
London W6 7PA
United Kingdom

Jones & Bartlett Learning books and products are available through most bookstores and online booksellers. To contact Jones & Bartlett Learning directly, call 800-832-0034, fax 978-443-8000, or visit our website, www.jblearning.com.

Substantial discounts on bulk quantities of Jones & Bartlett Learning publications are available to corporations, professional associations, and other qualified organizations. For details and specific discount information, contact the special sales department at Jones & Bartlett Learning via the above contact information or send an email to specialsales@jblearning.com.

The authors, editor, and publisher have made every effort to provide accurate information. However, they are not responsible for errors, omissions, or for any outcomes related to the use of the contents of this book and take no responsibility for the use of the products and procedures described. Treatments and side effects described in this book may not be applicable to all people; likewise, some people may require a dose or experience a side effect that is not described herein. Drugs and medical devices are discussed that may have limited availability controlled by the Food and Drug Administration (FDA) for use only in a research study or clinical trial. Research, clinical practice, and government regulations often change the accepted standard in this field. When consideration is being given to use of any drug in the clinical setting, the healthcare provider or reader is responsible for determining FDA status of the drug, reading the package insert, and reviewing prescribing information for the most up-to-date recommendations on dose, precautions, and contraindications, and determining the appropriate usage for the product. This is especially important in the case of drugs that are new or seldom used.

Production Credits
Executive Publisher: Christopher Davis
Editorial Assistant: Sara Cameron
Associate Production Editor: Laura Almozara
Associate Marketing Manager: Katie Hennessy
Manufacturing and Inventory Control Supervisor: Amy Bacus
Composition: Appingo
Cover Design: Kristin E. Parker
Cover Image: © Image Club Graphics
Printing and Binding: Malloy, Inc.
Cover Printing: Malloy, Inc.

Library of Congress Cataloging-in-Publication Data
Macenka, Deanna Glass-
   Johns Hopkins patients' guide to brain cancer / Deanna Glass-Macenka and Alessandro Olivi.
      p. cm. — (Johns Hopkins patients' guide to)
   Includes bibliographical references and index.
   ISBN-13: 978-0-7637-7425-7
   ISBN-10: 0-7637-7425-1
   1. Brain—Cancer—Popular works. I. Olivi, Alessandro. II. Title: Brain cancer.
   RC280.B7M324 2012
   616.99'481—dc22

                                                                    2010036985

6048

Printed in the United States of America
15 14 13 12 11   10 9 8 7 6 5 4 3 2 1

Dedication

This book is dedicated to all the newly diagnosed brain cancer patients and their families. Our hope is that this book will serve to educate and prepare you for the journey ahead of you. If we can help lessen the load and make your journey even a little bit easier by empowering you with knowledge and support, then we have succeeded in meeting our goal.

Deanna Glass-Macenka, RN, BSN, CNRN

Alessandro Olivi, MD

Contents

Contributors

Jaishri Blakeley, MD
Assistant Professor of Neurology, Oncology, and
    Neurosurgery
Director, The Johns Hopkins Hospital Comprehensive
    Neurofibromatosis Center
The Johns Hopkins Hospital
Baltimore, MD

Eileen Bohan, RN, CNRN
Assistant Professor of Neurosurgery, Department of
    Neurosurgery
The Johns Hopkins Hospital
Baltimore, MD

Henry Brem, MD
Harvey Cushing Professor of Neurosurgery
Chairman, Department of Neurosurgery
The Johns Hopkins Hospital
Baltimore, MD

Gary R. Shapiro, MD
Chairman, Department of Oncology
Johns Hopkins Bayview Medical Center
Director, Johns Hopkins Geriatric Oncology Program
The Sidney Kimmel Comprehensive Cancer Center at
    Johns Hopkins
Baltimore, MD

PREFACE

The diagnosis of cancer is, by itself, shell-shocking news to patients and their families. Learning that you have brain cancer could be even more unsettling given the significant unknowns associated with this diagnosis. Is my cognitive function going to be impaired? How can I cope with a possible neurological deficit? Will I have to endure brain surgery? All of a sudden your life is totally different, and you need help—lots of help.

Deanna Glass-Macenka and I have been involved in the initial care of many patients affected by brain tumors and with this book, we want to provide as much information as possible so you can be assisted in the course of your best treatment plan. Being educated about the different types of brain tumors and prepared about the next treatment step will be critical in assisting you in making sound and informed decisions.

Some brain tumors, specifically gliomas, are very different from other types of cancer. They have an inherently variable biological behavior, and the individual response to therapies may also vary greatly. That is why having an informed approach at all times toward the different treatment options is fundamental in maintaining an appropriate and beneficial positive attitude in spite of the initial striking diagnosis.

This book is the result of many years of practice in dealing with patients with newly diagnosed brain tumors. The information provided does not apply to all our patients but should be read, entirely or selectively, as a source of support during your individualized treatment plan. The book also provides resource information about the multidisciplinary team that will be dedicated to your care throughout this journey. The most troubling feeling that we have observed in our patients affected by brain tumors is the frequent unsettling feeling of not knowing what to expect. That is why we believe that educating our patients about all the resources available during their complex treatment course will hopefully be beneficial.

Our team is dedicated not only to the assistance of the patients that are initially struck with this diagnosis but also to the relentless quest to develop new and more effective forms of treatment for our future patients.

We know how incredibly difficult the times are that you and your family are going through and that you are probably living through the most challenging time of your life. We do not want you to feel alone in this, and our team will be assisting throughout this challenging journey.

Alessandro Olivi, MD

Introduction

How to Use This Book to Your Benefit

The goal of this book is to help you learn more about your cancer and make informed decisions about your care. By being better informed, we hope that you will be better prepared to confront the challenges ahead as you proceed through treatment and recovery. You will receive a lot of information from your healthcare team and will probably search the Internet or bookstores. No doubt friends and family members who mean well will attempt to give you advice about what to do and when to do it, and they will try to steer you in certain directions.

Your doctor has told you that you have brain cancer—words that you wish that you had never heard said about you. Even after hearing such news it is important to take the time to empower yourself with accurate information so that you can participate in the decision making about your care and treatment.

There is a natural sense of urgency to proceed with some type of treatment as soon as possible when you have a diagnosis of brain cancer. However, the initial decision you make about where to receive treatment and from which multidisciplinary team can be crucial in determining the overall treatment outcome. This book will give you the tools you need to make the informed decisions about your glioma brain tumor.

This book is designed to be a guide that takes you through the various treatment options and side effects and will help you put together a plan of action so that you can be a brain cancer survivor. The book is broken down into chapters that contain information about current surgical, radiotherapeutic, and systemic (chemotherapy) therapeutic options; combined modality treatment options; and recommendations for living with and surviving brain cancer.

There is also an index in the back and resources listed for your further review and education. This information will help you understand the how, when, and why of treatment options so you are in a much better position to be able to make treatment decisions with your doctors. Let's begin now with understanding what has happened and what the first steps are to getting you well again.

CHAPTER 1

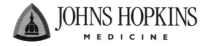

FIRST STEPS—I'VE BEEN DIAGNOSED WITH A BRAIN TUMOR

You have recently undergone some type of radiological examination and been told by a physician that you have a brain tumor and it's likely cancerous. This news can be quite overwhelming. Knowing what to do, where to go, and the "right" questions to ask are key in making sure you receive the best care possible. To start, let's discuss some basics.

BRAIN TUMOR BASICS

A brain tumor is a group of cells that has grown uncontrollably. Primary, or intrinsic, brain tumors originate in the brain and rarely spread to anywhere outside of the brain or spine (central nervous system).

PRIMARY BRAIN TUMORS

There are more than 120 types of primary brain tumors. In the United States, approximately 45,000 new cases of primary brain tumors are diagnosed each year. For the purpose of this book and all related discussions, we will focus on the largest group of primary brain tumors, called gliomas. Today, most medical institutions use the World Health Organization (WHO) grading system to classify brain tumors. The WHO classifies brain tumors by cell origin and cell behavior, from the least aggressive (benign) to the most aggressive (malignant). Some tumor types are assigned a grade. Factors that determine the tumor grade include how fast the cells are growing, how much blood is supplying the cells, whether dead cells are present in the middle of the tumor (necrosis), whether the cells are confined to a specific area, and how similar the cancerous cells are to normal cells. There are variations in grading systems, depending on the tumor type. The classification and grade of an individual tumor help predict its likely behavior.

Gliomas are divided into four grades, from the least aggressive (indolent) to the most aggressive (malignant or cancerous). Unlike tumors in many other parts of the body, gliomas can form in one of two ways: They can start as low grade (grade I or II) and over years become more aggressive, eventually becoming cancerous grade III or IV gliomas; or they can manifest very quickly, originating as high-grade cancerous tumors (grade III or IV). The hierarchy of gliomas, from the least aggressive and potentially curable (grade I) to the most malignant and incurable (grade IV), is as follows:

Low grade:

Grade I: Pilocytic astrocytoma

Grade II: Diffuse/infiltrating astrocytoma; oligo-dendroglioma

High grade:

Grade III: Anaplastic astrocytoma; anaplastic oligodendroglioma

Grade IV: Glioblastoma multiforme

Again, this book is devoted to the care and management of the largest group of primary brain tumors: gliomas, specifically high-grade malignant gliomas that encompass grades III and IV. Each year in the United States more than 17,000 people will be diagnosed with a malignant high-grade glioma.

CAUSES OF BRAIN TUMORS

The cause of brain tumors is unknown. Environmental and genetic factors may rarely cause some brain tumors, but no specific causative factors have been identified to date. No links have been found between gliomas and smoking, diet, cellular phones, or electromagnetic fields. Individuals who have received previous treatments with ionizing radiation to the head appear to be at a slightly increased risk for developing brain cancer at a later time.

Other factors associated with an increased incidence of gliomas include:

Sex. Men are slightly more likely to have gliomas than women.

Age. Those older than 50 years are more likely to have a glioma.

Ethnicity. Asians, Caucasians, and Latinos have a higher risk of developing a glioma.

Certain genetic disorders: Having Tuberous Sclerosis, Neurofibromatosis, Li-Fraumeni Syndrome, Turcot Syndrome, or Von Hippel-Lindau Disease can increase your risk of developing a glioma

Having a low-grade brain tumor. This can develop into a higher-grade tumor.

SYMPTOMS OF BRAIN TUMORS

The most common symptoms include headaches; seizures or convulsions; difficulty thinking, speaking, or finding words; personality changes; weakness or paralysis in one part or one side of the body; loss of balance; vision changes; confusion and disorientation; and memory loss. Different parts of the brain control different functions, so symptoms will vary depending on where the tumor is located in the brain.

A brain tumor takes up space within the skull, which is why it can interfere with the normal functions of the brain. A tumor can cause damage by increasing pressure in the brain, shifting the brain, and/or invading and damaging nerves and healthy brain tissue. The location of a brain tumor influences the type of symptoms people may experience. Diagnosing the presence of a brain tumor is the first step in determining a course of treatment.

DIAGNOSING A BRAIN TUMOR

A brain tumor diagnosis usually involves several steps. Something, whether it was headaches, a seizure, a head injury, or some other neurologic symptom, caused your physician to suspect a problem within your brain and, consequently, to order imaging. The imaging revealed an abnormality that appeared suspicious for a brain cancer. Your physician may have ordered further evaluative methods, including a detailed neurologic examination and additional brain imaging.

A neurologic examination is a series of tests to measure the function of the patient's nervous system. If the patient's responses to the exam are not normal, a brain scan may be ordered and the patient may then be referred to a neurologist or neurosurgeon for further evaluation.

The main methods of imaging the brain are computerized axial tomography (CAT) and magnetic resonance imaging (MRI). These scans use a contrast agent (or contrast dye), which is a liquid injected into a vein that flows into brain tissue. The difference in dye levels can show the difference between normal and abnormal brain tissue. Abnormal or diseased brain tissue may absorb more dye than normal, healthy tissue.

CAT scan (also referred to as CT scan) combines sophisticated X-ray and computer technology to show a combination of soft tissue, bone, and blood vessels. CAT images can determine some types of tumors, as well as help detect swelling, bleeding, and bone and tissue calcification. Usually, iodine-based contract agents are used during a CAT scan. People who are allergic to iodine should tell their doctor before having a CAT scan. People with kidney disease also should discuss the risk of this dye with their doctor. This is often the first scan used, especially in the case of emergency.

MRI is a scanning device that uses magnetic fields and computers to capture images of the brain on screen and on film. It does not use X-rays. It provides pictures from various planes, or visual "slices" of the brain, that can be combined on-screen to create a three-dimensional image of the tumor. MRI detects signals emitted from normal and abnormal tissue, providing detailed views of the brain anatomy and any areas of abnormality. MRI is currently the best available imaging for brain tumors, and you will likely have these scans done on multiple occasions to monitor your brain. The contrast material used for MRI scans is called gadolinium and is not iodine-based. People with kidney disease, however, should still discuss the risk of this dye with their doctor.

Ultimately, although malignant gliomas have very specific radiological characteristics, the only way to diagnose brain cancer for sure is to examine a piece of the tissue under a microscope. Tissue can be obtained in several ways. Biopsies are generally recommended if lesions are located deep within the brain and when an attempt at removal would cause irreversible damage to the surrounding brain. Resection, which is the surgical removal of suspected cancerous brain tumors, is always the preferred option, provided it can be performed without causing damage to the brain structure in the surrounding areas. Either way, the tissue sample will provide information on the types of abnormal cells present in the tumor.

GETTING TO KNOW THE BRAIN: ITS PARTS AND THEIR FUNCTIONS

The essential components of the central nervous system (CNS) are the brain and spinal cord. Malignant gliomas, which occur mainly in the brain, can, in very rare instances, spread to the spinal cord.

THE SKULL

The skull is a framework of 8 cranial and 14 facial bones that protect the brain. The cranium, the part of the skull that covers the brain, is made up of four major bones: the frontal, occipital, sphenoid, and ethmoid bones. There are four other bones in the cranium: two temporal bones, which are located on the sides and base of the skull, and two parietal bones, which fuse at the top of the skull. The areas where the bones in the skull meet are called sutures.

THE BRAIN

The brain is a soft, spongy mass of nerve cells and supportive tissue. The brain is responsible for the generation of the signals that control the neurologic function of the body. It has six main divisions: the frontal, parietal, temporal, and occipital lobes; the brain stem; and the cerebellum. In the center of the brain are four connected hollow spaces called ventricles. The ventricles contain a clear, waterlike liquid called cerebrospinal fluid (CSF) that circulates throughout the CNS. By surrounding the brain and spinal cord, the CSF cushions and protects these structures against injury. The CNS has a closed circulatory fluid system that drains into the bloodstream.

THE MENINGES

Three protective membranes—layers of tissue called meninges—surround the brain and spinal cord. The outermost layer, the dura mater, is a thick, leatherlike membrane. The second layer, the arachnoid mater, and the third layer, the pia mater, are thin membranes.

BRAIN FUNCTION

To understand your brain tumor fully, it is important to understand the different lobes and structures of the brain and their functions. See Figure 1 for information about the structures of the brain and their functions.

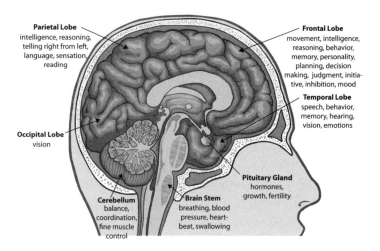

Figure 1   Brain Functions

Source: © Oguz Aral/ShutterStock, Inc.

LEARNING ABOUT YOUR DISEASE AND ITS PROGNOSIS

Gliomas account for almost 50% of all brain tumors diagnosed in the United States each year. Approximately 17,000 new high-grade malignant gliomas will be diagnosed this year in the United States. The median age of onset is 50 years, and men are affected slightly more frequently than women. There is no traditional staging system for primary malignant gliomas like there is for other primary cancers (e.g., breast, lung, etc.). This is because traditional cancer staging is based not only on the size of the tumor but also its invasion of surrounding tissues, and its spread to lymph nodes and distant organs. Gliomas rarely if ever spread outside the brain or CNS and by definition, gliomas infiltrate the surrounding tissue. There are, however, many factors that can impact the prognosis of a person diagnosed with a high-grade malignant gliomas, as listed here.

Age. Although the median age of onset is 50, those diagnosed at an earlier age tend to do better in terms of tolerating treatment and increased survival.

Overall health. Those patients who are in general better health with lack of other comorbidities such as diabetes, heart and lung disease, etc., tend to do better.

Location. The location of the tumor is an extremely important prognostic indicator. When a tumor is located in an area of the brain that is not essential for normal activities (a "non-eloquent area"), more of it can be removed without affecting one's neurological function.

Maintenance of neurological function. Patients who are able to maintain high-level neurological function tend to tolerate treatment better and have fewer complications, such as pneumonia and deep vein thrombosis.

Early detection and surgical resection. Although somewhat controversial, there is significant evidence to support that aggressive surgical resection using state-of-the-art techniques can improve patient outcomes and sustain longer survivals by safely removing as much tumor as possible and therefore decreasing residual tumor (tumor burden).

MGMT status. MGMT is a biomarker for a DNA repair enzyme found in gliomas. Research has shown that patients who have "methylation" of their MGMT are more susceptible to standard alkylating chemotherapy agents used in treating high-grade malignant gliomas (e.g., Temozolomide and BCNU [carmustine], to be discussed later in Chapter 3).

The median survivals, however, are still poor. Median survival for a patient with grade IV glioblastoma multiforme is about 12 months, and median survival for a patient with grade III anaplastic astocytoma is about 24 months.

TREATMENT OPTIONS

A variety of therapies are used to treat brain cancer. The type of treatment recommended depends on the size, type, and location of the tumor; its growth rate; and the general health of the patient. Treatment options include surgery, radiation therapy, and chemotherapy, or a combination of these. We will discuss each of these options in detail in subsequent chapters.

SELECTING A TREATMENT TEAM
AND MEDICAL CENTER

After your doctor diagnoses you with suspected brain cancer, he or she may refer you to one of several specialists. A team of healthcare providers will work with you throughout your treatment process. Specialists who treat brain cancer include neurosurgeons, medical oncologists, and radiation oncologists. If available at your treatment center, seek out neurosurgeons that have had specialty training or fellowships in brain cancer and that subspecialize in your specific kind of tumor (for example, neuro-oncologists only treat patients with brain or CNS cancer and neuro-radiation oncologists only treat patients with brain or spinal cancer). When choosing a neurosurgeon, look for one who has completed a tumor fellowship and/or is a brain tumor specialist. At larger centers, these physicians often act as a collaborative team. You should ask your primary care provider for advice in selecting an appropriate physician, preferably one at a cancer or brain tumor center, if possible.

Additional information is available from your local medical society, hospital, or medical school. You can also call (800) 4-CANCER to learn about National Cancer Institute-supported treatment centers located near you or receive a list of qualified doctors through the American Board of Medical Specialties (http://www.abms.org/).

You are the most important member of your healthcare team. Your situation is unique, and your treatment will be tailored to meet your needs. Play an active role during your therapy. Start by learning as much as possible about brain cancer. Most importantly, you should do the following:

- Be involved in the decisions that affect you.

- Learn about your cancer and your treatments in ways that feel right to you.

- Talk to your healthcare team about your worries or concerns.

- Keep your doctor, clinic, and hospital appointments.

- Ask your healthcare team how you can contact them between appointments if you have questions that need to be answered quickly.

GATHERING RECORDS

Your cancer specialist will want to review all of the medical records associated with your disease. You should bring copies of them with you to your visit and always keep an original copy for your own records. You may need to sign an authorization for the release of information before any records are released; you can do this in person, by mail, or via fax. Be sure to include all records, including those that contain details about the events that led up to your suspected diagnosis, such as office notes, emergency room records, and hospital discharge summaries. You will also need original radiology studies on film or on CD as well as the written report. Operative and pathology notes should be included if you have had any prior brain surgery or biopsy. If you had a biopsy performed at another institution, your current treatment team will likely ask for the original pathology slides to be reviewed by their own pathology team in order to confirm the diagnosis before a treatment plan is put into effect. You will have to request that these samples be sent.

All of these records will enable your healthcare team to make the best possible treatment recommendations for you. Many cancer centers require that this information be faxed and reviewed before an appointment date is given, so be sure to start gathering these records immediately to expedite the process.

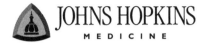

CHAPTER 2

MY TEAM—MEETING YOUR TREATMENT TEAM

Now that you have been given the preliminary presumptive diagnosis of brain cancer, the next step is to assemble a brain cancer oncology or neuro-oncology team. This team contains many healthcare professionals, all with a common goal—to help you get well and stay well for as long as possible. Each member has a specific role related to brain cancer and its treatment. The following is a list of the major members of your team:

- *Neurosurgical Oncologist*. This is a neurosurgeon who specializes in brain tumors and performs the brain cancer surgery—needle biopsy, open biopsy, or craniotomy for removal/debulking of your brain tumor. The neurosurgical oncologist is a subspecialist who does additional training in dealing with tumors of the CNS. This is often the first specialist you see.

- *Neuro-radiation Oncologist.* This doctor specializes in the treatment of cancer patients by using the delivery of radiation to the CNS. This consultation is initiated by your neurosurgeon and usually occurs 1 to 2 weeks after your surgery when the final pathology results are available. The radiation oncologist works closely with the neurosurgical and medical oncologists in designing your treatment plan. In many cases, patients with brain cancer receive chemotherapy in conjunction with radiation therapy.

- *Neuro-radiologist.* This is a radiologist who has completed an additional fellowship or training in studying and diagnosing images of the brain, head, neck, and spine.

- *Neuro-oncologist/Medical Oncologist.* This is someone who specializes in brain cancer and selects the medicines for your systemic treatment. This doctor is either a medical oncologist specializing in brain cancer or a neurologist who has completed additional fellowship training in oncology. He or she specializes in treating cancer with chemotherapy or targeted therapies aimed at stopping your tumor recurrence. This physician is often a patient's main doctor along the continuum of care and often helps to coordinate care given by other specialist. The consultation to see this doctor often occurs about two weeks after your surgery has been completed when the final pathology results are available; it is initiated by the neurosurgeon who performed your surgery. Neuro-oncologists work closely with neurosurgical oncologists in designing your treatment plan.

- *Neurologist/Epileptologist.* Some patients with brain tumors experience seizures. If you are affected by seizures, you may need to see a neurologist who specializes in seizure management. In addition, neurologists may be very helpful in the assessment of neurological deficits.

- *Pathologist/Neuropathologist.* Although you will probably never meet this physician, the pathologist is a very important member of your team. He or she will examine the tissue from your tumor under a microscope to determine the grade of your tumor and other valuable prognostic information. In some cases, pathologic information can be used to design patient-specific treatments. Some centers have a neuropathologist who specializes in the study and diagnosis of brain and CNS disease.

- *Nurses.* You will meet many nurses as you progress along your journey through each phase of your treatment, beginning with surgery, chemotherapy, and radiation. Often, each of your physician specialists will have his or her own nurse available to you. Patient education, patient/family support, assessment of your clinical needs, administration of chemotherapy, and ongoing evaluation of your progress are some of the essential functions nurses perform.

- *Social Worker/Patient Liaison.* This is someone who specializes in offering support as well as addressing financial concerns you may have. These individuals will be available to you both during your stay as an inpatient and when you are receiving outpatient therapies.

- *Survivor Volunteer.* Many cancer centers offer emotional support from survivor volunteers who have completed their treatment of brain cancer and want to provide one-on-one support to newly diagnosed brain cancer patients. They can provide a candid view of what to expect and can be a great support along your journey. Also inquire about brain cancer support groups held at your treatment center, as they provide invaluable support and education to brain cancer patients and their families.

YOUR INITIAL APPOINTMENT AT A CANCER CENTER

At this point, you have undergone imaging of your brain, whether because of recent symptoms or perhaps because you have suffered your first seizure. This imaging revealed what you have been told is likely a malignant tumor that has originated in your brain. The first doctor you will need to meet in consultation at the cancer center is a neurosurgical oncologist. Some general neurosurgeons may also manage patients with brain cancer. It is important to know the credentials, board certifications, and volume of brain cancer patients they treat. You want a neurosurgeon who performs brain cancer surgeries often.

Be sure that whomever you speak with at the cancer center knows that you have been newly diagnosed with a brain tumor, which you have been told may be cancerous. He or she should be able to expedite your appointment with one of the center's specialists. Your recent diagnosis is very scary; you may feel that it is an emergency and you need to be seen today. The truth is that if you have already been seen by a doctor who has reviewed your imaging and potentially placed you on some medications, such as steroids for swelling and maybe even seizure medications if you need them (see pages 37–39 for more information), you will need a timely, but not necessarily urgent, appointment with a neurosurgeon. If your cancer center has a Web site, take this time to check it out; learn about their brain cancer program, and read the biographies of their specialists so you can make some choices about which providers you want on your team.

Make sure you get the exact address and clear directions for your appointment. This information can often be found on the cancer center's Web site. Also inquire about the exact time of the appointment and parking recommendations. If you have never been to the facility before, allow yourself extra time to get there just in case you hit traffic or get lost. Being late for your first appointment will frustrate you and just add to the stress in your day. If possible, arrive a little early to familiarize yourself with the office. This will allow you to complete any necessary forms, review insurance information, and simply sit and relax for a moment. Take a deep breath and if you haven't already done so, and write down a list of questions that you want covered during your appointment.

Now comes the frustrating part. You have arrived in time for your appointment, yet you may have to wait because your provider is delayed. Try to remember that many of the patients being seen by your physician this day may have also been urgently added to the schedule in the last week or so and have recently been diagnosed with potential brain cancer, just like you. When it is your turn, your provider will give his or her complete attention to you and will devote whatever time is needed to explain treatment recommendations and discuss your questions and concerns.

WHAT TO BRING WITH YOU FOR YOUR FIRST CONSULTATION

You have your appointment and directions. Hopefully the person who scheduled your appointment went over what to bring, but in case he or she was not clear or you want a refresher, here are some guidelines to follow. These recommendations will help to make your appointment as productive and efficient as possible:

- *Imaging studies.* Be sure to bring any imaging pertaining to your potential diagnosis of brain cancer. This means the results of all brain MRIs, MRI spectroscopy, CAT scans, and any other radiographic tests that you may have had. The facility where you had these studies done will provide you with either hard copies of the films or the images on a CD, along with the radiology report. More than likely, your surgeon will ask to keep the studies so they can be reviewed with other team members, such as a neuroradiologist, or presented at a tumor board meeting. Occasionally, your neurosurgeon will request that the studies be repeated due to less than optimal quality. Your films can often be electronically uploaded to your cancer center's database for surgical planning and ongoing evaluation. There may be a charge associated with this service, so be sure to discuss it with your provider. You may have been told by the facility where you had your studies performed that the films need to be returned in a predetermined amount of time. This is not true. Do not let these statements worry you. They are technically your property. Let the surgeon's office staff handle the inquiries about the returning of films.

- *Pathology report/slides.* If you have not had any brain surgery yet, then this section does not apply to you. In some cases, patients have undergone biopsies or less than total removal of their brain tumors at outside facilities. They are now seeking a second opinion to see if more tumor can be removed. If so, it is likely that your surgeon will request that you have the pathology report as well as the actual pathology slides. The surgeon may request that they be delivered prior to the appointment so his or her neuropathologist can render an opinion about the accuracy of the information provided in the typed report. This information and the accuracy of the first pathology sample will assist your surgeon in making recommendations to you as well as aid in surgical planning.

- *Copies of your medical records.* It is likely that some of your medical records were required in order for you to get an appointment at your cancer center. This is usually done by the referring physician's office. This information is useful and may include office visit notes pertinent to your diagnosis, emergency room notes, and hospital discharge summaries if you have had any inpatient admissions related to your diagnosis. Operative notes should be included if you have had any surgeries related to your diagnosis. Records that include names, doses, and instructions for any medications you have been placed on are also important to bring to this visit. It is a good idea for you to make copies of all of these records for yourself to avoid delaying any other visits that may require this information.

- *Insurance information.* You were likely required to give your insurance information to the person who scheduled your appointment; however, be sure to bring all necessary cards to your appointment to confirm that all information is correct. Speak with your insurance provider ahead of time to determine whether the provider you have chosen is in-network and what your estimated copayments will be, if any. If a cancer diagnosis is suspected or confirmed, additional assistance or case management is available to you to make sure you get all the support you need in a timely manner. Also, ask the neurosurgeon if he or she wants you to have additional radiological studies. If they need to be preauthorized, can they be performed at your chosen treatment center or must they be done by an outside provider?

WHO TO BRING WITH YOU FOR YOUR FIRST CONSULTATION

Bring a trusted family member or friend along with you. When individuals are stressed, they often only hear and retain part of what has been said. A lot will be discussed at this visit with your neurosurgeon, and you may feel overwhelmed and have difficulty keeping it all straight. The person you bring can act as a scribe to write down exactly what was said for you to review later. You may also want to bring along a tape recorder. Most doctors are comfortable with their discussions being recorded.

OTHER CONSIDERATIONS FOR YOUR FIRST CONSULTATION

Be sure to bring an accurate list that includes the following information:

- Any other surgeries you have previously had

- Medical conditions that you are currently being treated for (hypertension, diabetes, etc.)

- Medications you are taking, including any vitamins, minerals, herbal supplements, and over-the-counter medications (such as aspirin)

- Any drug or food allergies you may have

- Your family medical history, including cancers, heart disease, lung disease, and other serious illnesses

If you are uncertain of your family medical history, get help obtaining this information from another family member.

Many centers will send you a questionnaire ahead of time for you to complete and bring to the appointment. This questionnaire will include all of the information just covered. If your cancer center has a Web site, often the questionnaire can be downloaded for your completion. If not, you will be given one when you arrive for your appointment and asked to complete it prior to being seen.

QUESTIONS TO ASK AT YOUR FIRST CONSULTATION

Preparing a list of questions in advance to ask your neurosurgeon can be helpful in making the visit as efficient as possible. However, you should be provided with contact information, so if you forget to ask questions or if you think of new ones, you should be able to have your questions addressed. The following list should help you get started:

1. What kind of brain tumor do you suspect I have?

2. What grade of disease do you suspect I have based on what you know so far from my history and imaging studies?

3. Am I a candidate for surgery? Will it be a resection (removal) or a biopsy, and why? How much of my tumor do you think you can surgically remove?

4. If applicable: Did your pathology team confirm the accuracy of my biopsy or previous resection results? Do you have a neuropathologist and will he or she be reading my pathology?

5. How soon will my surgery be scheduled?

6. What educational material or information do you offer to prepare me for surgery, and what should I expect?

7. Will you shave my head?

8. Where and how big will the incision be?

9. Is the center known for its treatment of brain tumors?

10. How long will I be hospitalized after my surgery?

11. Does the hospital have a neuro-ICU and staff for postsurgical care?

12. How much pain will I be in after surgery?

13. What will my activity level be after surgery? What will I be able to do and not do?

14. Who will be my contact here for any questions I may have? Is there an emergency number for this practice after hours?

15. Do you have any education material for family members?

16. How many brain cancer surgeries do you perform each year? (As a guide, the number of brain cancer surgeries the neurosurgeon performs should be at least 50% of his or her practice, and the physician group he or she works with should do a combined 300 cases a year).

17. Can I meet other patients who are going through something similar? What support groups are available?

18. Regarding available technology: What specialized equipment is available in the operating room? Is there a computer navigation guidance system? An operating microscope? An intraoperative ultrasound? An intraoperative MRI?

19. If I am interested in additional therapy at the time of surgery (e.g., Gliadel wafers, discussed in Chapter 3), is it available to me?

20. When will I be able to return to work or my normal activities? Will I need help at home or someone to stay with me? Will I need to go to an inpatient rehabilitation center or outpatient physical therapy? If so, what are my options?

21. Who else will be involved in my care and when will I meet them?

22. Do you regularly attend tumor boards to present cases for team discussion?

23. Do you work with a multidisciplinary team of oncologists who specialize in brain cancer?

24. How soon after surgery will I see a medical and/or radiation oncologist?

25. Do you anticipate that I will need chemotherapy? If so, why?

26. Do you anticipate that I will need radiation? If so, why?

27. What side effects might I expect from treatment? Are there any special precautions I will need to take, or medications I will need to reduce side effects?

28. What will my life be like during and after treatment? What kind of quality of life can I expect?

29. How often will I see you after surgery for ongoing evaluation?

30. Who will coordinate my care? Do you have a contact person to help me with scheduling appointments as well as help me navigate my brain cancer treatment?

31. How are subsequent appointments arranged for me and when do these happen?

32. If my tumor recurs, will I be treated at the same facility or transferred to another center?

Even if you already know some of the answers, the questions are still worth asking as a way to obtain more complete information and to spark a dialogue with your doctor. Open, honest, and thorough discussions between you, your family, and your healthcare team will facilitate decision making and help make it easier to address challenges that may occur.

ADDITIONAL TESTS YOU MAY NEED

Most brain tumors that originate in the brain—specifically malignant gliomas—rarely, if ever, spread outside the CNS. Therefore, unlike other cancers, scans of the rest of the body are generally unnecessary.

Your surgeon will review all of your imaging studies to determine if any additional ones are required before the surgery. If your tumor is near your speech center, which for most of the general population is controlled in the left side of the brain, a functional MRI (fMRI) may be performed. This special MRI requires patients to speak, read, and follow commands during an MRI. These tasks require extra blood to be sent to the parts of the brain responsible for the specific function. fMRIs measure the blood flow and provide images outlining these "functional" areas. These images will assist your surgeon in planning and performing your resection. Your surgeon will use these images in the operating room to help guide the removal of tissue not essential for normal activities and preserve those areas of your brain that are functional.

Additionally, the day before or morning of your surgery, you may be required to undergo a special MRI. Special stickers called fiducials will be placed on your forehead and temples and behind your ears. You will then have an MRI. A special computer program used in the operating room creates three-dimensional intraoperative pictures using the fiducials as references. This process is called intraoperative neuronavigation. The computer program will help guide your neurosurgeon in resecting as much tumor as is safely possible and will help him or her to identify tumor when it may not necessarily look abnormal to the naked eye.

Blood tests are not helpful in the management or diagnosis of brain cancer. However, your surgeon will order some as part of the routine preoperative evaluation. You may also need a chest X-ray and electrocardiogram. These tests are not related to your brain tumor; rather, they are requirements for anyone having an operation. The preoperative evaluation can be performed by your primary care physician or internist or can be arranged at the hospital where your surgery will be performed. This evaluation is necessary to make sure you are in optimal condition to receive anesthesia.

CONTACTING YOUR TEAM MEMBERS

Request business cards from each healthcare provider you meet, and ask what their office procedures are for responding to questions or concerns you may have. Usually there is one contact person whose role it is and whom you can rely upon to address your questions. Find out if you can communicate with any of the team members by e-mail. If you have a question, take the time to evaluate your thoughts and, if need be, write them down so you do not forget them and are ready when you speak to your provider.

NAVIGATING APPOINTMENTS

Ask what the process is for appointment scheduling, obtaining test results, scheduling for your surgery, seeing a neuro-oncologist and a radiation oncologist after your surgery, and addressing any other clinical needs that may arise. In some centers, your point person may be a nurse or an office manager in the physician's office; in other centers, it may be someone who is called a navigator or case manager.

FINANCIAL IMPLICATIONS OF TREATMENT AND INSURANCE CLEARANCE

Being diagnosed with a cancerous brain tumor was never in your plan. There is never a good time to get this disease, and hearing the diagnosis alone has no doubt caused you a great deal of stress and anxiety. If you are employed outside the home, you will likely need to take a leave of absence to undergo surgery as well as radiation and chemotherapy. Getting your "ducks in a row" early will help to decrease anxiety in the long run. Finding out how much sick time you have accrued, your employer's long- and short-term disability coverage, copayment information, prescription coverage, and other medical expense issues is helpful in planning your budget, which may be changing for a while. Your insurance company may require referrals to see specialists, have tests performed, and undergo surgery and other authorized treatments. If you need help figuring this all out, ask for a social worker to assist you. Many cancer centers have financial assistants specially trained to help their patients. Don't be afraid to ask.

You may be offered the opportunity to enter a clinical trial associated with brain cancer. Some insurance companies may cover their members and the costs associated with clinical trials, and others may not. If you are interested in a trial, the research nurse/coordinator will help you with determining your coverage.

If you do not have health insurance, there are resources available to patients who need help and meet certain criteria for financial assistance and coverage of their cancer treatment. Check with the social worker at the cancer center where you are being treated to get assistance and referrals. There are also organizations that provide financial support for transportation to and from treatment, food for you and your family, and coverage of some medications. They are not available in all states, so ask the social worker exactly what is available in your geographic area. Financial support services are often not well advertised. You or a family member will need to take the initiative to ask about them instead of waiting for someone to tell you about them. Money is often one of the primary reasons family members get into arguments, so avoid this conflict by discussing all these issues up front. Plan ahead and be proactive in asking to meet with the social worker to discuss what support services are available to you.

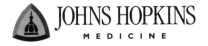

CHAPTER 3

TAKING ACTION—COMPREHENSIVE TREATMENT CONSIDERATIONS

This chapter is dedicated to explaining the various types of treatment for high-grade gliomas and the decisions involved in making the best choices for you. The management of this disease usually begins with surgery, either a biopsy or resection, followed by radiation along with chemotherapy. To help further elucidate standard treatment regimens for high-grade malignant gliomas, the National Comprehensive Cancer Network (NCCN) Practice Guidelines have been summarized in Table 1.

The NCCN is an international alliance of the leading cancer centers whose goal is to improve both the effectiveness and the quality of the care that patients receive. NCCN works to achieve this by developing resources and clinical practice guidelines for patients, clinicians, and others in health care.

Table 1 Standard Guideline for Treatment of Anaplastic Gliomas/Glioblastomas

RADIOLOGIC PRESENTATION	TREATMENT PLANNING	CLINICAL IMPRESSION	SURGERY	LOCAL THERAPY
MRI suggestive of Anaplastic Glioma (Anaplastic Astrocytoma–AA/ Anaplastic Oligodendro-glioma–AO) or Mixed Anaplastic Oligoastrocytoma (AOA) or GBM (Glioblastoma Multiforme) *Also gliosarcoma	Multidisci-plinary input (neuro-surgery, neuro-oncology, neuro-radiology, radiation oncology) for treatment planning if feasible	Maximal safe surgical removal is possible	Maximal safe removal with residual enhancing tumor	± carmustine (BCNU) wafer (chemo chips)
			Complete removal of enhancing tumor confirmed by intra-operative neuronaviga-tional imaging *intra-operative patho-logical confirmation of diagnosis must sup-port high-grade glioma (AA/AO/AOA/GBM)	
		Maximal safe surgical removal not feasible	Stereotactic biopsy or Open biopsy or Subtotal removal	Carmustine (BCNU) not indicated

Adapted with permission from the *NCCN Clinical Practice Guidelines in Oncology (NCCN Guidelines™) for Central Nervous System Cancers V.1.2011.* © 2011 National Comprehensive Cancer Network, Inc. All rights reserved. The NCCN Guidelines™ and illustrations herein may not be reproduced in any form for any purpose without the express written permission of the NCCN. To view the most recent and complete version of the NCCN Guidelines, go online to NCCN.org. NATIONAL COMPREHENSIVE CANCER NETWORK®, NCCN®, NCCN GUIDELINES™, and all other NCCN Content are trademarks owned by the National Comprehensive Cancer Network, Inc

Table 1 Continued

Tests/ Evaluation	Pathology		Patient Functional Status	Adjuvant Treatment	Follow-Up
MRI as soon as clinically stable (preferably within 72 hours) after surgery to establish extent of resection and new baseline	Anaplastic Gliomas (AA/AO/AOA) or **Anaplastic gliomas; consider 1p19q analysis		Good Performance status: Evaluation using functional scales Karnofsky Performance Scale (KPS ≥ 70)	Fractionated external beam (conventional) Radiation Therapy (RT) or Chemotherapy or Combined Chemo and radiation	MRI 2–6 weeks after completion of RT, then every 2–4 months for 2–3 years, then if stable may perform MRI less frequently
			Poor Performance status (KPS < 70)	Fractionated external beam RT (standard or decreased) or Chemotherapy or Best supportive care	
	GBM (Glioblastoma Multiforme)	Treated with carmustine (BCNU) wafers	Good Performance status	Fractionated external beam (conventional) Radiation Therapy (RT) ± concurrent and adjuvant temozolomide	
		No carmustine (BCNU) wafers	Poor Performance status (KPS < 70)	Fractionated external beam RT (standard or decreased) or Chemotherapy or Combined treatment or Best supportive care	

When an MRI suggests a high-grade malignant glioma, the NCCN recommends consultation and treatment at a center where an experienced multidisciplinary team, including a neurosurgical oncologist, neuro- or medical oncologists, and neuro- and radiation oncologists are available for treatment planning. Treatments may include surgery, administration of chemotherapeutic drugs designed to kill cancer cells, and/or treatment in the form of radiation also designed to destroy cancer cells. Surgery should always be considered as the first treatment option if the tumor is in a location where it can be safely removed. During the operation, a sample of your tumor will be sent to pathology for examination (intraoperative frozen section). If this shows a high-grade malignant glioma (AO, AA, AOA, or GBM), your neurosurgeon will consider placing a BCNU wafer in the area of your brain where your tumor is located. If surgical resection is not safe based on the location of the tumor, a needle or open biopsy should be performed to confirm pathological diagnosis before any further treatment planning can begin. An MRI should be obtained within 72 hours of a resection to establish a new baseline and extent of residual tumor. Once the diagnosis is confirmed by a final pathology (and, if indicated, genetic marker) review, multidisciplinary treatment planning can continue. Treatment of anaplastic tumors (AA/AO) should include external beam radiation with or without concomitant (at the same time) chemotherapy. If a patient's general well being (performance status) is relatively good, aggressive treatment with daily external beam radiation along with oral chemotherapy may be considered. If the final pathology review shows a diagnosis of a glioblastoma or gliosarcoma, external beam radiation should be considered. Even if an intraoperative BCNU wafer was placed, additional chemotherapy with oral temozolomide should be considered, depending on age and if overall general wellbeing and health of the patient is adequate (see Chapter 10). An MRI should be obtained 2–6 weeks after radiation is completed. Oral temozolomide is generally given to high-grade malignant gliomas for at least 6 months (or cycles) provided that the patient has no serious side effects or evidence of progression of disease. MRIs are usually repeated every 2 months throughout the course of chemotherapy. After the completion of chemotherapy, scans are repeated every 2 months to monitor your condition. Each step of the NCCN guidelines will be explained in detail in the following paragraphs.

SURGERY

Surgery is often the first-line treatment for malignant gliomas. Just the thought of brain surgery for most individuals is overwhelming. Compound that with the news that the tumor found growing in their brain is likely cancerous and the fear factor multiplies. After all, our brain allows us to think, feel, understand, and interact with the world around us. Having part of our brain removed is an obvious threat to those abilities. Some patients have been diagnosed with low-grade gliomas in the past and now have had radiological changes that are suspicious of transformation to a higher grade; others have been newly diagnosed with a radiological abnormality thought to be brain cancer. Either way, the surgical decisions that will need to be made are similar.

BIOPSY VERSUS RESECTION

It is important to choose a neurosurgeon who is experienced and competent in operating on brain tumors. Experience is a difficult thing to quantify. At least 50%

of his or her practice should be brain tumors and/or the neurosurgical group should perform at least 300 brain tumor surgeries a year. The first decision is whether to have a needle biopsy, open biopsy, or a craniotomy for removal or resection of your tumor.

Biopsy

In general, biopsies are performed when tumors are located very deep within the brain or when they involve an "eloquent structure" (an area essential to normal activities), when an attempt at removing the tumor is thought to be associated with great risk for permanent damage to the brain likely causing significant neurologic impairment. Needle biopsies are performed using a computer-assisted intraoperative system and a long needle that is precisely placed into the brain; a tiny piece of your tumor is removed through this needle. Open biopsies are performed via a hole that is made in the skull through which a piece of the tumor is removed. In either of these biopsy methods, only a very small piece of the tumor is removed and sent to pathology for analysis. Due to the small amount of tissue removed, in a small number of cases, a diagnosis cannot be accurately determined.

Craniotomy

A craniotomy is an operation to open the skull (cranium) in order to access the brain for surgery. The goal of a craniotomy for tumor resection is to completely remove the tumor. If this is not possible, the goal is "debulking," or partial or subtotal resection (removing some of the tumor). In general, craniotomies are performed when tumors are located closer to or reaching the surface of the brain. They require that a piece of skull (called a bone flap) be temporarily removed to create a window through which your neurosurgeon can remove the tumor in a piecemeal fashion. Not only is there more tissue that can be sent for pathologic evaluation, but patients can often benefit from the resection or debulking of the tumor and decreasing the tumor burden. In lay terms, this means diminishing the amount of tumor cells left behind. This procedure can potentially improve symptoms (e.g., headaches, seizures, other neurologic impairments), and, in theory, the treatment that will follow (e.g., radiation, chemotherapy) will have less work to do.

In some cases, your neurosurgeon may recommend performing an AWAKE craniotomy. Although just the thought of this might be frightening, you need to know that this approach is becoming more widely used and, with modern techniques, is very well tolerated by the patients. It is indicated when important areas of the brain (functional centers such as speech and motor control) are in proximity or overlying the tumor mass. It is very helpful to the surgeon, in these cases, to have active cooperation of the patient to directly test all of these functions during the crucial portion of the operation so "mapping" and protection of those areas can be achieved. You also need to know that during the initial and last phases of the operation (the ones that can cause a degree of discomfort), you will be adequately sedated and will not feel any pain. During the central phase of the operation, however, you will be responsive and will be asked to perform simple tests such as naming objects, counting and recounting, or squeezing hands. Once again, the objective of this approach is to maintain your intact function while the tumor is aggressively removed. Your surgeon will be able to explain to you why it is advisable to have the procedure done this way and to provide you with the exact sequence of the different phases of the operation.

By definition, primary malignant gliomas are infiltrative, which means there are no clear borders separating the cancerous area from the surrounding brain. Microscopic extensions of cancerous brain often extend into the normal brain around and near the tumor. Sometimes these extensions are referred to as "fingerlike projections" or "tentacles." Therefore, even if the best neurosurgeon removes everything that looks abnormal, there are tumor cells left behind. It is impossible to remove 100% of a malignant glioma. A skilled and experienced neurosurgical oncologist will attempt to remove as much tumor as possible without permanently damaging any areas of the patient's brain that may result in loss of function (e.g., motor, speech, cognition). The goal of any tumor resection is to maintain or if possible improve neurologic function. For instance, if a patient has no deficits or impairment of neurologic function prior to surgery, then the goal should be to be as aggressive as possible during the tumor removal but maintain all of the patient's functions as they were prior to surgery. If a patient presents with a motor dysfunction (e.g., weakness, coordination), the goal should be to resect the tumor but not worsen the existing dysfunction. In some cases, patients who have motor, speech, or other problems prior to the resection may experience an improvement. This usually happens when the functional part of the brain is not directly affected by infiltration of cancerous tumor, but rather by pressure or swelling in the brain as a result of the tumor.

PRESURGERY MEDICATIONS

Your brain tumor may be causing pressure or swelling in your brain. It may also cause irritation that could lead to seizures. For this reason, you may have been placed on one or more medicines.

Antiepileptic Drugs

People with brain tumors may experience seizures related to their tumor, surgery, or the treatment they receive that can irritate the surrounding brain. Therefore, it is common for patients with brain tumors to require antiepileptic drugs (AEDs). AEDs are used to suppress the electrical activity in the brain that can lead to seizures. In general, AEDs are recommended around the time of surgery for a short duration; they may be permanently recommended for people who have had a history of seizures.

Some frequently prescribed AEDs are:

- Dilantin (phenytoin)
- Keppra (levetiracetam)
- Lamictal (lamotrigine)
- Tegretol (carbamazepine)
- Topamax (topiramate)
- Trileptal (oxcarbazepine)
- Depakote (valproic acid)

Your neurosurgeon and neurologist will determine which medication is best for you and how long you should take it. The following is some general information on these types of drugs. Please refer to the individual drug package insert and your pharmacist/healthcare team for more information specific to the drug you have been prescribed.

Dosage. Dosage varies, depending on the specific drug and each patient's needs. It is important not to skip doses. If you do forget a dose, take it as soon as you remember and then resume your normal schedule. If you have any questions, contact your healthcare provider.

Possible side effects. All AEDs can cause side effects. Some side effects do not depend on how long and how much you are taking; some do. People react differently. Common and/or important side effects are:

- Rash

- Confusion

- Lethargy

- Sleepiness

- Unsteadiness

Blood tests. Some AEDs require regular blood tests to monitor their therapeutic levels and your body functions.

Special considerations. Women have special issues regarding AEDs because of pregnancy, birth control pills, and breast-feeding. Women on AEDs should use birth control or speak with their medical team regarding plans for pregnancy.

Effects on ability to drive or use machines. Due to differing individual sensitivity, some people might experience sleepiness or other CNS-related symptoms, especially at the beginning of treatment or following a dose increase. Therefore, caution is recommended in those people when performing skilled tasks such as driving vehicles or operating machinery. Patients are advised not to drive or use machines until it is established that their ability to perform such activities is not affected by their medication and their seizures are well controlled.

The fact that you are on an AED does not automatically make you ineligible to drive a car. Each US state has guidelines and restrictions that are based on whether patients have ever had a seizure. Driving privileges may be awarded or revoked based on frequency of seizures and how much time has elapsed since the person last experienced a seizure. Consult your local department of motor vehicles for additional information.

Steroids

Your brain tumor may be causing pressure or swelling in your head. Therefore, you may need to take steroids to help control the swelling. The steroid most commonly used to treat swelling and edema in the brain is called Decadron (dexamethasone).

Dosage. Your doctor will tell you how much Decadron to take and how often to take it. Do not change the dose or schedule (how often you take the drug) without talking to your doctor. If you miss a dose, take it as soon as you can. Do not stop using this medicine suddenly without asking your doctor. You will need to taper (reduce the dose gradually) your use before stopping it completely.

Possible side effects. You may experience the following while taking Decadron:

- Increased appetite/weight gain. Limit your intake of salt and sugar to reduce the chance of this effect.

- Mood changes and/or difficulty sleeping.

- Muscle weakness, especially of the thigh muscles. Consider physical therapy.

- Increased blood sugar. Call your doctor if you have increased urination or thirst.

- Gastrointestinal bleeding. Call your doctor if you have black or tarry stools.

- Increased risk for infection. Avoid people who are sick. Call your doctor if you have fever or chills or are exposed to chicken pox or measles.

- Easy bruising and/or fragile, thin skin.

- Acne.

- Irregular menstrual periods.

- Possible joint pains.

Important information. Important notes related to Decadron use include the following:

- Take your steroids with food or milk to reduce the risk of an upset stomach.

- Make sure your doctors and pharmacists know all the other medications you are taking.

- It is important for you to take the doses as prescribed. If you are unable to take all your doses because of the flu or some other problem, call your doctor immediately.

- Decadron is an important medication; do not allow your supply to run out.

- Talk to your doctor before getting flu shots or other vaccines while you are on Decadron.

- When starting steroid therapy or changing the dose, it may take several days for you to feel the full effect of the change.

- Notify your doctor immediately if you have new or worsening headaches, nausea and/or vomiting, or any new symptoms.

PREPARING FOR SURGERY

Before your surgery, you should have a basic understanding about the procedure that will be performed and what recovery will be like. The recovery period will vary and depend upon what procedure is performed. Generally, the recovery from a biopsy is less than the recovery from a craniotomy for resection or debulking of your tumor. The recovery period also depends on your age and overall health prior to the surgery. Younger people tend to recover faster, as do people in good overall health prior to the surgery. Ask your surgeon about the average hospital stay and recovery for your planned surgical procedure. Other factors that can affect your recovery include whether you had any neurologic problems or deficits (e.g., numbness, weakness, speech or visual problems) prior to the surgery. These deficits may improve after a surgery but may temporarily worsen or be permanent. Be sure to discuss these possibilities with your surgeon so you understand your risks and suspected surgical prognosis.

The recovery period is a time when not only your incision, but also your brain is healing. You will be given a list of restrictions before your discharge that generally includes no bending, no strenuous activity or lifting of more than 5 pounds, no driving, and no alcohol. You will be instructed to be up and about, taking short walks throughout the day if you are able. Frequent rest periods will be needed. A well-balanced diet is recommended to optimize healing. Be sure to discuss caring for your incision with your surgeon before discharge.

OPERATIVE PROCEDURE

The general procedure for a craniotomy includes the following steps:

- A preoperative MRI is obtained either the day before or the day of your surgery and provides your surgeon with computer guidance or intraoperative neuronavigation in the operating room. This MRI involves placing small round stickers, called fiducials, on and around your head before entering the MRI scanner. These stickers need to remain on your head until you enter the operating room so be careful if they are placed the day before. Once you enter the operating room, the intraoperative guidance system is calibrated to provide your surgeon with surgical guidance during the procedure.

- In most cases, you are given a general anesthetic.

- A small strip of hair on your scalp is shaved; at some centers, a larger amount of your hair may be shaved.

- Your head is placed on a round or horseshoe-shaped headrest so that the area where the brain tumor is thought to lie is easily accessible. To restrict any head movement, your head is clamped into place with a head-pin-fixing device.

- Through preoperative imaging, the neurosurgeon determines the most appropriate site for the craniotomy. Once you are asleep, the procedure begins by cutting through the scalp. Small holes (burr holes) are drilled into the skull.

- An instrument is used to cut from one burr hole to the next, creating a removable bone flap.

- The membrane covering the brain (dura) is opened, exposing the underlying brain.

- The brain tumor is identified and resected.

- The dura is closed.

- After the operation is finished, the piece of excised bone is put back and held in place with tiny plates and screws (these are usually made of titanium and will not interfere with future MRIs, airport travel, etc.); the muscle and skin are stitched up.

- Sometimes it is necessary to place a drain inside the incision to remove any excess blood left from the surgery. This drain will be removed a day or two later.

The length of the craniotomy varies depending on the location of the tumor and the complexity of the case. Be sure to discuss the specifics of your situation with your neurosurgeon.

LOCAL THERAPY

Some patients diagnosed with high-grade gliomas may benefit from what is called local therapy. This treatment means that after the surgeon resects your tumor and an intraoperative pathology sample confirms high-grade malignant gliomas, the surgeon may place a treatment, in the form of chemotherapy (a drug aimed at killing cancer cells), directly into the cavity from which the tumor was removed. If your doctor thinks you may be a candidate, he or she should discuss this with you prior to surgery. You may also want to discuss this treatment with your neurosurgeon to see if local therapy is right for you.

Gliadel

The Gliadel wafer is a unique form of drug-delivery treatment for brain tumors. The wafers are small biodegradable polymer discs about the size of a dime. If the intraoperative pathology (frozen section) shows a high-grade glioma, Gliadel wafers may be placed during surgery, provided the tumor is solitary, does not cross the midline of the brain, and is located in the upper lobes (cerebrum) of the brain. The wafers (up to eight) are implanted into the tumor site; there, they slowly release a chemotherapy drug, BCNU. It takes only 3 to 4 minutes to place the wafers.

Each wafer contains a precise amount of BCNU. Over the next 2 to 3 weeks, the wafers slowly dissolve, bathing the surrounding cells with BCNU. The goal of the therapy is to kill any tumor cells that may have been left behind after surgery. Because the wafers are biodegradable and eventually dissolve, there is no need for another procedure to remove them.

The Gliadel wafer is the only chemotherapeutic implant approved by the US Food and Drug Administration (FDA) for use during neurosurgical resection, including at the time of the initial resection of newly diagnosed high-grade malignant gliomas and subsequent surgeries for recurrent glioblastoma multiforme.

Side Effects of Wafer Therapy

Chemotherapy can potentially cause side effects. Certain side effects reported with intravenous BCNU treatment have not been seen after implantation of Gliadel wafers. Side effects that have been reported in association with Gliadel wafers include seizures, pain, infection, and abnormal wound healing. Although these events may occur after brain surgery alone, they may occur more frequently when Gliadel wafers are used. In studies, the most common side effects reported, more often in patients receiving Gliadel wafers than in patients receiving placebo, included pain and abnormal wound healing.

Impact of Wafer Therapy on Other Cancer Therapies

Wafer therapy will not prevent you from undergoing any standard, nonexperimental treatments including other chemotherapies or radiation, but it may prevent you from participating in some clinical trials of unapproved compounds or from receiving experimental drugs (see pages 56–63). You and your physician should review the details of clinical trials you are considering to see if that is the case.

Contraindications to Wafer Therapy

If you have had a previous allergic reaction to BCNU, you should not receive the wafer. Make sure your doctor knows about this and any other allergies.

IMMEDIATELY AFTER SURGERY

After the operation, you can expect the following:

- You will probably be admitted to the intensive care unit. Some centers have special intensive care units dedicated to neurologic patients. You will likely be there at least one night and will then be transferred to a regular nursing unit when your condition is stabilized.

- As soon as the doctors and nurses have completed their assessments and you are stable, your family members will be allowed to see you. This usually takes about an hour.

- You will have intravenous lines and a heart monitor, as well as a catheter in your bladder.

- A loose-fitting mask may be placed over your mouth, which will deliver oxygen.

- You will also likely have a soft dressing on your head for a day or two.

- Your head will be elevated to about 30 degrees to reduce the risk of intracranial (inside the skull) pressure.

- You will be given pain medication as prescribed. You should not have a lot of pain. Most people just take Tylenol (acetaminophen) after the surgery. Let your nurse know if you have any pain or headaches. Your medications can be changed accordingly.

- The doctors and nurses caring for you will test your neurologic functions regularly. For example, they may examine your pupils with a flashlight, ask you simple questions, and ask you to perform simple tasks.

- Your eyes may be swollen and bruised.

- Expect to be out of bed, eating and starting to take short walks the day after surgery.

- You can expect to stay in the hospital for 2 to 5 days. The length of stay depends on many factors, such as the type of surgery you had and whether you experienced complications or required further treatment.

- Stitches or staples are usually removed 1 to 2 weeks after surgery.

- You should bring some comfortable clothes (a bathrobe, for example) to wear after surgery.

- Once you are eating and drinking normally, the intravenous lines will be removed from your arm.

The nurses will keep track of what you eat and drink as well as how much you urinate.

- After your surgery, your doctor may consult a physical therapist, occupational therapist, or speech language pathologist to help with your recovery. Your doctor and therapy team will work together with you to determine the best and safest discharge plan for when you leave the hospital.

POSTOPERATIVE IMAGING

A postoperative image should be performed before you leave the hospital. A CAT scan is usually sufficient for patients who have undergone a needle biopsy but MRIs are preferred for those patients who have undergone resection. In most cases, if clinically stable, the MRI should be obtained within 72 hours if possible. This allows the new radiographic baseline to be established and the ability to assess the extent of resection. After several days, scar or reactive tissue can form, which may cause enhancement and ultimately make it difficult to determine if there was any enhancing tumor remaining after the resection.

Final pathology results will take a week or two, but your neurosurgeon may discuss preliminary findings with you while you are still in the hospital. Once your brain cancer diagnosis has been confirmed, the next phase of your treatment will begin. As discussed in Chapter 3, because of the infiltrative nature of the tumor, further postoperative treatment is required to prevent or delay tumor recurrence. A referral or consultation request will be sent to both radiation and medical oncology by some member of your healthcare team. The standard treatment of newly diagnosed high-grade malignant gliomas (grade III anaplastic astrocytoma/anaplastic oligodendroglioma and grade IV glioblastoma multiforme) after biopsy or resection is radiation along with oral chemotherapy.

RADIATION THERAPY

External beam fractionated radiation therapy is the first line standard of care and should be considered in the treatment for all patients with pathologically confirmed high-grade malignant gliomas. Radiation therapy uses X-rays and other forms of radiation to destroy cancer cells. The energy of the radiation is absorbed by cancer cells, damaging their genetic material so that they are no longer able to grow. By planning the treatment carefully and delivering the radiation precisely, the oncologists and therapists can avoid irradiating normal healthy cells. Because X-rays are light energy, they pass through the human body and can be used to treat cancers that are deep inside the body or located in areas that may be hard to reach through surgery. Radiation therapy uses advanced technology to create high-energy, or short-wavelength, beams to treat cancers.

Your first visit to radiation oncology will be for a consultation. The radiation oncologist will perform a physical examination and document your health history. He or she will then develop tailored recommendations for radiation therapy. If you accept the recommendations, you will then be scheduled for a treatment planning session.

The treatment planning session is administered using a device called a simulator. Your radiation treatment planning begins with the simulation scan. The radiation therapist will custom fit a positioning mask, and a CAT scan will be taken of your head. These scans are used to create X-ray images of your brain and pinpoint the exact location of the tumor. The images are then used to create a three-dimensional picture of your brain anatomy. Once computer images have been obtained, the physician uses sophisticated computer applications to design a radiation treatment course, which includes the radiation dose and how best to deliver it. The radiation oncologist will give the treatment plan to a dosimetrist and/or a medical physicist, who will then create radiation calculations. Treatment calculations include the level of radiation energy to be applied (i.e., the dose), the angle of the treatment beam, and the amount of time for a given beam. The calculations are given to the radiation oncologist for approval or changes. Once all the specialists agree, you will be scheduled for the treatment sessions. This process usually takes about a week.

Radiation therapy treatments are usually given in small portions of the total prescribed dose, known as fractions. These fractions are usually administered every weekday over a period of several weeks (usually 5 to 7 weeks). Most treatment visits take between 15 and 45 minutes; the actual treatment time is only a few minutes. Each daily dose or treatment is called a fraction. Most people *do not* experience any physical sensation during treatment. Your radiation treatments *do not* make you radioactive. Radiation is cumulative, which means you may experience more side effects during the last few weeks of treatment. Each treatment is administered by a certified radiation therapist who monitors your progress.

SIDE EFFECTS OF RADIATION

Radiation treatment can affect normal cells and may produce a variety of side effects depending on the amount of radiation given and the size and location of the area treated. The common side effects of radiation treatment to the brain are due to swelling of the tissue in and around the tumor or tumor bed. They include, but are not limited to, the following:

- *Fatigue.* Mild fatigue is a common side effect of radiation therapy. A nap during the day, if necessary, should restore your energy levels. Treatment-induced fatigue usually resolves within 4 to 8 weeks after treatment. If you experience persistent, excessive fatigue or decreased consciousness, tell your radiation team.

- *Headache.* Radiation-related brain swelling can cause headaches, which should be reported to your radiation team, especially if you have headaches in the morning or headaches associated with nausea and vomiting or worsening neurologic symptoms, or if the headaches you have now are more severe or more frequent than the ones you had before treatment. If you are taking Decadron, continue to do so as prescribed, but it is likely that the dosage will need to be adjusted; changing the dose can quickly ease symptoms.

- *Nausea and vomiting.* These symptoms may indicate significant brain swelling, which may require an increase in your steroid dose. Steroids can also cause stomach upset, and often medications are prescribed to settle the stomach.

- *Changes in sensation and movement.* Tell your doctor right away if you experience any of the following: a change in vision, hearing, or speech; a change in the feeling in the face, trunk, arms, or legs; an abrupt change of bowel or bladder habits; weakness of the arms or legs; unsteady walk; seizure or "blackouts"; or any other changes. You may require changes in your medication.

- *Loss of hair.* Hair follicles are very sensitive to radiation. You will likely see hair loss from the area being irradiated 2 to 3 weeks after the start of radiation. This may be temporary (with regrowth usually occurring within 3 to 6 months) or permanent, depending on the amount of radiation you have received. Check to see if the cancer center has an image recovery center of some sort. If available, this center can help you with things such as selecting a wig, tying a scarf, and determining what kind of skin care regimen would work best for you.

CHEMOTHERAPY

Chemotherapy refers to drugs (chemicals) that are used to destroy cancer cells. It is used to attack cancer cells and stop their growth. Chemotherapy may be used alone or in combinations of drugs. It is used to treat fast-growing, aggressive, or malignant tumors; it is sometimes used to treat slower-growing, less aggressive tumors as well.

Chemotherapy drugs are carried in the blood and reach cells all over the body, including healthy cells. Chemotherapy not only damages the rapidly dividing cancer cells but also other cells in your body that normally divide rapidly such as hair follicles, bone marrow, and the cells that line the digestive tract. Damage to these normal cells is what often causes the many side effects. Side effects are usually temporary and will often gradually disappear when the treatment is over. However, chemotherapy side effects can be severe and can interfere with treatments, so you should report any side effects to your doctor or nurse.

Chemotherapy may work by stopping cells from dividing or by blocking proteins that a tumor cell's DNA needs to survive. Brain cancers are especially difficult to treat with chemotherapy because of the brain's specialized protective mechanism called the blood–brain barrier, an adaptation of the circulatory system in the blood vessels that supply the brain. The capillaries that are normally responsible for supplying oxygen and nutrients to the brain have especially tight junctions that limit the substances allowed to pass into the brain. This is especially helpful at preventing bacteria and other substances that could cause damage from entering the brain, but it can also prevent many chemotherapeutic substances from entering as well. Therefore, the blood–brain barrier makes many chemotherapeutic agents less effective in the CNS. Not all tumors are sensitive to chemotherapy; therefore, each patient and each tumor type are considered individually. Your physician will discuss which options are appropriate for you.

ADMINISTRATION OF CHEMOTHERAPY

Chemotherapy can be given in one of four ways:

1. *Intracavitary administration.* Your neurosurgeon can implant chemotherapy-impregnated wafers directly into the cavity from which your tumor was removed. (Refer to the section on Gliadel wafers on page 44.)

2. *Intravenous administration.* The drugs can be given directly into your veins via a needle either by direct injection or continuous infusion.

3. *Oral administration.* The drugs can be given in pill form.

4. *Intrathecal administration.* The drugs can be infused directly into your CSF.

SIDE EFFECTS OF CHEMOTHERAPY

The risks associated with this form of treatment vary depending on the type of chemotherapy given. Generally, some common side effects associated with chemotherapy include:

- Nausea and vomiting

- Diarrhea or constipation

- Weight loss

- Loss of appetite and/or taste alterations

- Fatigue

- Numbness or tingling in hands or feet

- Hair loss

- Rash, acne, itching, or burning skin

- Dry mouth and/or mouth sores

- Pain

- Bone marrow suppression: Bone marrow activity is decreased and causes decreased formation of red and white blood cells as well as platelets

  - Anemia (low red blood cell count): fatigue

  - Thrombocytopenia (low platelet count): blood clotting difficulty, bruising

  - Neutropenia/Leukopenia (low white blood cell count): increased risk of infection

These side effects will be discussed further in Chapter 4.

RADIATION AND CHEMOTHERAPY

The radiation care team will prescribe, plan, and monitor your radiation treatments. The standard of care for patients with high-grade malignant gliomas (grade III anaplastic astrocytoma/anaplastic oligodendroglioma and grade IV glioblastoma multiforme) is to receive oral chemotherapy at the same time, or "concurrently," with a drug called TMZ (temozolomide). TMZ is an oral alkylating chemotherapy agent, which means it damages DNA and triggers tumor cell death. This treatment schema is well established in the brain cancer community and is often referred to as the "Stupp protocol" (because it is based on well-known and established research by Dr. Roger Stupp). Around the same time, a consultation with a medical oncologist or neuro-oncologist will occur. The process, goals, risks, and side effects will be discussed during your consultation.

Your oncologist will assess whether TMZ might be useful to you. Generally, this treatment will begin at the start of radiation therapy. Prescriptions for TMZ pills as well as chemotherapy instructions and education should be given to you at this visit. Some centers may even have special classes that you attend. You will likely need some baseline blood work completed at this visit as well.

TMZ chemotherapy is dosed by your weight, and you will take it every day, including weekends, from the first to the last day of radiation therapy, for up to 49 days. You will be asked to take it approximately 1 to 2 hours before your scheduled daily radiation treatment and in the morning on weekends or nontreatment days (e.g., holidays). Anti-nausea drugs will also be prescribed. During the course of radiation, you will likely have visits with the radiation and/or medical oncology care providers every week to monitor for side effects of the treatment and medications associated with the treatment. At these visits, you will likely be asked to continue to give samples of your blood to monitor for side effects of the treatment.

Make sure you have phone numbers and instructions to contact your providers both during office hours and after hours and on weekends should you require urgent attention.

It is also a good idea to make sure that your primary care physician and/or internist are kept informed of your treatment plan. Give this doctor's name and contact information to your radiation and medical oncologists so they can keep him or her informed of your treatment plan. This will be helpful should you require this doctor's services at any time during your treatment.

After your radiation with concurrent TMZ treatments have been completed, you will be given an approximate 4-week break. Provided that you have had no serious complications and that your blood counts remain stable, you will be instructed to resume your TMZ chemotherapy. This time, however, your dosing will likely be increased and you will only take it for 5 days in a row. The next 23 days you will take no chemotherapy. Each 28-day period is called a "cycle." You will continue to have your blood monitored every week or two until your oncologist tells you to stop. Generally, between every two cycles of chemotherapy, a new MRI of your brain will be performed to evaluate the effects of your treatment. This schedule usually continues for at least 6 months or 6 cycles, but your oncologist should discuss the treatment plan with you.

CLINICAL TRIALS

Clinical trials, also called research studies, test new treatments in people with cancer. The goal of this research is to find better ways to treat cancer and help people who have cancer. Many types of treatment are tested in this way, such as new drugs, new approaches to surgery or radiation therapy, new combinations of treatments, or new methods such as gene therapy, vaccination, immunotherapy, etc.

A clinical trial is one of the final stages of a long and careful research process. The search for new treatments begins in the laboratory, where scientists first develop and test new ideas. If an approach seems promising, the next step may be testing a treatment in animals to see how it affects cancer in a living organism and whether it has harmful effects. Of course, treatments that work well in the lab or in animals do not always work well in people. Studies are done with cancer patients to find out whether promising treatments are safe and effective. Without clinical trials, doctors could not improve the treatment of brain cancer, nor could ways be developed to prevent it in the future. Your doctors may at any time during your treatment discuss with you the opportunity to participate in a clinical trial. Be open-minded and listen carefully to the details of the study.

WHY CLINICAL TRIALS ARE IMPORTANT

Clinical trials are important in two ways. First, cancer affects us all, whether we have it, care about someone who has it, or worry about getting it in the future. Clinical trials contribute to knowledge and progress in treating cancer. If a new treatment proves effective in a study, it may become a new standard treatment that can help many patients. Many of today's most effective standard treatments are based on previous study results. Clinical trials may also answer important scientific questions and suggest future research directions. Because of progress made through clinical trials, many people treated for cancer are now living longer.

Second, the patients who take part may be helped personally by the treatment(s) they receive. They get up-to-date care from cancer experts, and they receive either a new treatment being tested or the best available standard treatment for their cancer. Of course, there is no guarantee that a new treatment being tested or a standard treatment will produce good results. New treatments also may have unknown risks. But if a new treatment proves effective or more effective than standard treatment, study patients who receive it may be among the first to benefit.

There are many different kinds of clinical trials. They range from studies focusing on ways to detect, diagnose, treat, and control brain cancer to ways that address quality-of-life issues that affect patients with brain cancer. Most clinical trials are carried out in phases. Each phase is designed to learn different information and then build upon the information previously discovered. You may be eligible for studies in different phases, depending on the current status of your disease, anticipated therapies planned for you, and treatments you have had already. You will be monitored very closely at specific time points while participating in a clinical trial.

THE THREE PHASES OF CLINICAL TRIALS

Each phase answers different questions about the new treatment.

- *Phase I trials* are the first step in testing a new treatment in people. In these studies, researchers look for the best way to give a new treatment (e.g., By mouth, intravenous drip, or injection? How many times a day?), try to find out if and how the treatment can be given safely (e.g., What is the best dose?), and watch for any harmful side effects. Because little is known about the possible risks and benefits in phase I, these studies usually include only a small number of patients.

- *Phase II trials* focus on learning whether the new treatment has an anticancer effect (e.g., Does it shrink a tumor? Does it improve blood test results?). As in phase I, only a small number of people take part because of the risks and unknowns involved.

- *Phase III trials* compare the results of people taking the new treatment with results of people taking standard treatment (e.g., Which group has better survival rates? Which group has fewer side effects?). In most cases, studies move into phase III testing only after a treatment shows promise in phases I and II. Phase III trials may include hundreds of people around the country. Comparing similar groups of people taking different treatments for the same type of cancer is another way to make sure that study results are real and caused by the treatment rather than by chance or other factors. Comparing treatments with each other often shows clearly which one is more effective or has fewer side effects.

NONTHERAPEUTIC CLINICAL TRIALS

Many patients want to participate in a clinical trial and make a difference in our understanding of brain cancer and the treatments used, but do not necessarily want to receive a new investigational treatment or drug. Nontherapeutic clinical trials involve monitoring some aspect of a patient's health throughout the course of his or her care without adding a new investigational agent to the patient's current treatment.

YOUR RIGHTS, YOUR PROTECTION

Before and during a cancer treatment study, you have a number of rights. Knowing them can help protect you from harm. Some of your rights are as follows:

- Taking part in a treatment study is up to you. You have the right to know what alternative treatments are available (both standard therapy and clinical trials), and to choose one of these instead of the study that is being presented to you.

- If you do enter a study, doctors and nurses will follow your response to treatment carefully throughout the research.

- If researchers learn that a treatment harms you, you will be taken off the study right away. You may then receive other treatments.

- You have the right to leave a study at any time.

One of your key rights is the right to informed consent. Informed consent means you must be given all the facts about a study before you decide whether to take part. This disclosure includes details about the treatments and tests you may receive and about their possible benefits and risks. The doctor or nurse will give you an informed consent form that goes over key facts. If you agree to take part in the study, you will be asked to sign this informed consent form.

The informed consent process continues throughout the study. For instance, you will be told of any new findings regarding your clinical trial, such as new risks. You may be asked to sign a new consent form if you want to stay in the study. Signing a consent form does not mean you must stay in the study. In fact, you can leave at any time. If you choose to leave the study, you will have the chance to discuss other treatments and care with your own doctor or a doctor from the study.

ELIGIBILITY FOR CLINICAL TRIALS

Each study has its own guidelines for who can participate, called eligibility criteria. Generally, participants in a study are alike in key ways, such as the type and stage of cancer, age, gender, or previous treatments. The eligibility criteria are included in the study plan. To find out if you are eligible for a particular study, talk to your doctor, or the doctor or nurse in charge of enrolling patients in the study.

PROS AND CONS

While a clinical trial is a good choice for some people, it may not be the best option for others. Consider the following possible benefits and drawbacks. You may want to discuss them with your doctor and the people close to you.

Possible Benefits

- Clinical trials offer high-quality cancer care, and you may be among the first to benefit from a new treatment approach.

- By looking at the pros and cons of clinical trials and your other treatment choices, you are taking an active role in a decision that affects your life.

- You have the chance to help others by improving cancer treatment.

Possible Drawbacks

- New treatments under study are not always better than, or even as good as, standard care. They may have side effects that doctors do not expect or that are worse than those of standard treatment.

- Although a new treatment may have benefits, it may not work for you. Even standard treatments, which have been proven effective for many people, do not help everyone.

- Health insurance and managed care providers do not always cover all patient care costs in a study. What they cover varies by plan and by study. The doctor, nurse, or social worker involved in the study will check with your insurance company prior to your enrollment in the study.

COSTS OF CLINICAL TRAILS

Many times, the group sponsoring the trial will cover the cost for things like experimental drugs and other expenses directly associated with the trial. However, there may be some other costs indirectly associated with the trial that are not covered. Even if you have health insurance, your coverage may not include some or all of the associated costs. This is because some health plans define clinical trials as "experimental" or "investigational" procedures. However, they may be willing to pay if the trial treatment is similar to a standard treatment. Because lack of coverage for these costs can keep people from enrolling in trials, the National Cancer Institute is working with major health plans and managed care groups to find solutions. Regardless, a coordinator working on the specific study should contact your insurance company prior to enrollment to determine your benefit coverage. Ask to speak with this person and also speak directly with your insurance company so you are well informed of your financial responsibilities before you enroll.

OTHER QUESTIONS YOU MAY HAVE
ABOUT CLINICAL TRIALS

The following is a list of questions that you may find helpful when considering enrollment in a brain cancer clinical trial.

1. What is the purpose of this study?

2. How many people will be included in this study?

3. What does the study involve?

4. What are my alternatives to participating in this study?

5. What kind of tests and treatment will I have?

6. How are the treatments given and what side effects might I expect?

7. What are the risks and benefits of the protocol?

8. Has anyone enrolled so far seen any benefits? If so, what benefits?

9. How long will the study last?

10. What type of long-term follow-up care is provided for those who participate?

11. Will I be responsible for any of the costs associated with this trial? Will my insurance company pay for any of this?

12. When will the results be known?

Realize that many brain cancer patients derive substantial benefits from participating in clinical trials. The treatment you have already received likely started as a clinical trial years ago. Participation can therefore benefit you. Perhaps equally as important, you may be contributing in a major way for the next patient dealing with this disease.

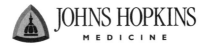

CHAPTER 4

BE PREPARED—THE SIDE EFFECTS OF TREATMENT

P atients undergoing treatment for brain cancer experience various side effects. These side effects may result from the treatment or from some of the commonly used medications used to control brain swelling and seizures in patients with brain tumors. Some side effects are easily controlled and others are more difficult. This chapter discusses some of the more common side effects of the medications as well as the radiation and/or chemotherapy that you may encounter. Be sure to discuss these side effects with your oncology team as they apply to your individual treatment plan. This chapter is not intended to scare or overwhelm you, but rather to arm and prepare you for issues that may occur and need to be addressed during your treatment. It will also educate you and make you aware of things to look out for.

SIDE EFFECTS OF STEROIDS

Brain tumor patients, especially those with high-grade malignant gliomas, are often required to take steroids—namely, Decadron—to help control the edema and swelling in their brain caused by the tumor, surgery, radiation, or chemotherapy (see Chapter 3 for more on Decadron). Treatments are all aimed at killing the tumor cells, which in turn can cause more edema in your brain. Therefore, steroids may become a part of your daily regimen and may be necessary throughout some or all of your treatment. Steroids have their own unique set of side effects and for some are difficult to tolerate. Great care will be taken by your healthcare provider to use only enough steroids to control your cerebral edema so that your side effects can be minimized.

Side effects may be induced quickly and include:

- Difficulty sleeping
- Increased sweating
- Increased appetite
- Nervousness/agitation
- Mood changes/swings
- Indigestion
- Dizziness
- Blurry vision

Long-term side effects may include:

- General body discomfort, joint or muscle pain, and/or muscle weakness
- Puffing of the face
- Weight gain
- Redistribution of fat

Always take your steroid dose with food to minimize any gastrointestinal irritation. If sleeplessness occurs, discuss an alternative dose schedule with your physician so that several hours will elapse between your last dose of the day and your bedtime.

As with any medications, be sure to discuss any new or prolonged side effect with your physician.

SIDE EFFECTS OF ANTIEPILEPTIC DRUGS

Most brain cancer patients are required to take AEDs for at least short periods of time during their disease process. If you have never had a seizure, you may only be required to take an AED around the time of surgery (see Chapter 3); others will require seizure medication for longer periods of time or even indefinitely. Each seizure medication has its own individual set of side effects. The more common side effects include the following:

- Drowsiness/sleepiness
- Fatigue
- Poor coordination/unsteadiness
- Behavior changes
- Attention difficulty
- Loss of appetite/nausea/vomiting
- Tremors
- Blurred or double vision
- Clumsiness

Many of these symptoms may improve with time and others may not. Be sure to discuss your tolerance of the medication with your physician, as there are many options that may be a better fit for you.

NON-SPECIFIC TREATMENT SIDE EFFECTS

COGNITIVE DYSFUNCTION

People receiving radiation or chemotherapy often complain about problems with memory (e.g., forgetting names, losing their keys). As a brain tumor patient, you have even more reason to have difficulty with cognition: You have a tumor in your brain that has just been operated on, you are completing or have completed brain radiation, and you are likely receiving chemotherapy all within a short period. It is certainly understandable if your brain is not working at its best. You may experience difficulty paying attention, finding the right words, remembering things, or learning new things. These effects can begin soon after treatment has started or may not appear until much later. They do not always go away. Any symptoms you may have had prior to starting your treatment (weakness, memory, speech problems) may in fact get worse during this time as well. Be sure to discuss any changes with your oncology team, as increasing your steroids or manipulating your AEDs may help.

The following techniques can help to heighten memory and concentration:

- *Jot down lists or tasks.* Write down in a notebook or calendar each task you must perform and how long it will take; also write down the time and location of any appointments. Plan your whole day and be realistic about what you can accomplish in one day. Refer to these notations frequently throughout the day to help stay on track or to refresh your memory with important information.

- *Set up reminders.* Place small signs around the house to remind you of things to do, such as lock the door.

It is also a good idea to set up a flow sheet with your medications listed by day, dose, and time. Be sure to cross off each dose as you take it so you don't repeat or miss one. Pill organizers are often helpful in staying on schedule with your medications.

- *Manage stress.* Minimizing stress may help improve your memory and attention.

- *Review what you plan to say.* Before you go to a doctor appointment, family event, or work function, write a list of questions you want to ask, concerns you want to discuss, names and dates you want to remember, and/or key points you want to make. Take notes with you and review.

- *Repeat what you want to remember.* Saying things several times in your mind may help you to remember and hold onto information longer.

These symptoms may become quite severe and may or may not improve with time. Your doctor or nurse can also make formal referrals to occupational and speech therapists, who specialize in these areas and can evaluate your symptoms and provide more focused and structured therapy. Most importantly, enlist the help or your family and support system to take over some of the tasks that seem difficult for you (e.g., balancing the checkbook).

ANXIETY

Anxiety is a normal response to new or stressful situations. It is common for people with brain tumors to experience symptoms of anxiety. In addition, the brain tumor itself or the therapies used to treat it can alter brain chemistry. The medications used to treat brain tumors (e.g., steroids) can also cause anxious feelings. Anxiety can make brain tumor symptoms or treatment-related side effects more intense. If you think you may have symptoms of anxiety, it is helpful to tell your medical team; they can help you.

Common symptoms of anxiety include:

- Nervousness

- Tension

- Fear

- Restlessness

- Irritability

- Difficulty concentrating

- Insomnia

At times, feelings of anxiety can become overwhelming and lead to panic attacks. Symptoms of panic attacks include:

- Shortness of breath or the feeling of choking

- Shaking or tremors

- Racing pulse

- Sweating or hot, flushed face

- Feelings of losing control or dying

It is important to talk about your feelings and concerns; doing so is part of your total well being. Along with loved ones and friends, staff can help you manage your anxiety. Let your medical team know if you are experiencing anxiety, especially if you have panic attacks. The medical team can evaluate your current medications and treatments to see if they may be causing anxiety. The medical team also can assist you in contacting social workers, psychiatric nurses, psychiatrists, and clergy who can help. There are many options for treating your anxiety, including counseling and therapy, relaxation exercises or guided imagery, and safe and effective medications.

DEPRESSION

Depression is common in patients with brain tumors. Often depression and anxiety occur together. Symptoms of depression include:

- Feelings of persistent hopelessness

- Feelings of helplessness, worthlessness, or uselessness

- Feelings of deserving punishment or inappropriate guilt

- Inability to enjoy life or experience pleasure

- Desire to harm oneself

- Changes in appetite, sleep, energy, or the ability to concentrate not directly related to treatment side effects

Becoming upset or feeling "fed up" when dealing with a major illness such as a brain tumor is normal. It is common to have a down mood, especially when experiencing the stress and symptoms of cancer (e.g., pain, headache) or the many side effects related to cancer treatment (e.g., fatigue, nausea/vomiting, diarrhea). Some medications, such as steroids, used to treat brain tumors or treatment side effects can affect a person's mood. Most people, however, note an improvement in their mood as symptoms and side effects are managed or go away. As suggested for coping with anxiety, it is important to talk about your feelings and concerns; doing so is part of your total well-being. There are trained professionals—social workers, nurses, psychiatric nurses, psychiatrists, clergy, physicians—on staff to listen to you and help with emotional problems during these stressful times. They can offer a variety of treatments, including counseling, therapy, and safe, effective medications for treating depression.

You can access professional help by doing any of the following:

- Talk with the members of your medical team (physicians, nurses, and social workers) about your feelings and concerns.

- Request to talk with a psychiatric liaison nurse.

- Contact your insurance company's mental health service, and ask for a referral to a mental health professional who has experience working with people who have cancer.

Seek professional help immediately if:

- You are thinking of hurting yourself.

- You are thinking about suicide.

- You have a history of depression and are experiencing the symptoms listed earlier in this section.

ANEMIA

Anemia by definition is an abnormally low level of red blood cells (RBCs). RBCs contain hemoglobin (an iron protein) that provides oxygen to all parts of the body. If your RBC level is low, parts of your body may not receive all the oxygen that they need to function well. Anemia can be caused by the loss of blood related to recent surgery or as a result of radiation or chemotherapy, which can be toxic to RBCs and inhibit RBCs from replenishing themselves as they normally would. Patients with anemia often report feeling tired or fatigued. In severe cases, the fatigue may interfere with the individual's quality of life. Other symptoms of anemia may be headache, light-headedness, dizziness, activity intolerance, or shortness of breath. You should notify a member of your oncology team immediately if you experience any of these symptoms.

Your provider can prescribe medications (e.g., Epogen or Procrit [epoetin alfa] and Aranesp [darbepoetin alfa]) to help stimulate the production of RBCs and raise your blood cell count. Oral iron supplements can also help treat anemia. Unfortunately, neither of these options works instantly. In fact, they require several weeks to establish the full effect; therefore, in some cases, you may require a blood transfusion to restore your blood levels if they are dangerously low.

THROMBOCYTOPENIA: LOW PLATELETS

Platelets are the component of your blood responsible for blood clotting. Patients with low blood platelet counts (thrombocytopenia) are at risk for spontaneous bleeding, easy bruising, and excessive bleeding after minor trauma. Chemotherapy can commonly cause low platelet counts. Be sure to report any bleeding or bruising to your provider immediately. If you are in fact experiencing a low platelet count, avoid any activity that may cause bleeding until your counts improve. Activities to avoid may include playing sports, shaving with a razor other than an electric one, flossing your teeth, or walking barefoot. Aspirin and ibuprofen can also increase your risk for bleeding, so be sure to discuss these medications with your provider before taking them. In severe cases, you may be prescribed a platelet transfusion if your levels remain at a low level or you show signs of bleeding.

INFECTION

People with cancer are often at risk for various infections. This risk may be linked to steroids that they have been on to control the swelling in their brain. Steroids lower the body's ability to fight infection and may mask the signs of an infection. Chemotherapy may also put individuals at risk for developing infections. The same treatments they are undergoing to fight and destroy cancer cells can often weaken their immune system. When harmful bacteria, viruses, or fungi enter the body and the body is not able to destroy them, an infection occurs. Symptoms including fever; chills; sweating; a sore throat; mouth sores; pain or burning during urination; diarrhea; shortness of breath; a productive cough; and swelling, redness, or pain at an incision site may indicate that an infection is present. There are several important things you can do to help lower your risk for acquiring an infection, including:

- Frequent hand washing

- Brushing your teeth at least twice a day

- Avoiding crowds of people

- Completely cooking your food (especially eggs and meat), and thoroughly washing fruits and vegetables

Family members or friends you see frequently should get flu shots to help reduce the risk of infection, and, of course, you should avoid contact with anyone who currently has an infection or virus of any kind. If you experience any symptoms or are concerned that you may be developing an infection, take your temperature. Contact your provider immediately for a fever greater than 100.5°F, or any other signs of infection. A visit and more testing (i.e., blood test, urinalysis, chest X-ray, etc.) may be necessary to determine if you need antibiotics or even admission to the hospital.

NAUSEA AND VOMITING, AND TASTE/APPETITE ALTERATIONS

Nausea and vomiting are a common side effect of many, but not all, chemotherapy agents. Some patients may experience alterations in their ability to taste, and foods that were previously enjoyable are no longer tolerable. Pain medications, too, have been known to contribute to nausea. Anorexia, or loss of appetite, often occurs. The complete inability to eat, weight loss, or even dehydration can result and may even require hospitalization. High-caloric, nutritionally balanced beverages are available and can be purchased in most grocery stores. Nausea/vomiting can be managed with medication, so be sure to discuss these symptoms with your provider so he or she can address them. Changes in what and how you eat may also be useful in managing these symptoms and include the following suggestions:

- Follow directions given by your provider on whether to eat or not before you take or receive your chemotherapy.

- When you do eat, be sure to eat small amounts. Small, frequent, light meals often are better tolerated than large ones.

If nauseated:

- Bland foods and liquids often work best.

- Eat dry crackers.

- Limit the amount of fluids you take with your meals. This will prevent overextending your stomach, which will make nausea worse.

- Maintain adequate liquid intake between meals. Try to stick to clear liquids such as water, apple juice, herbal tea, or bouillon.

- Avoid foods with strong odors.

- Avoid fatty, greasy, and fried foods.

- Avoid spicy foods, alcohol, and caffeine.

- Eat foods that are cool or at room temperature. This will keep aromas at a minimum and help to decrease nausea.

- Suck on peppermint candies, and use peppermint-flavored lip balm.

If experiencing taste alterations, you may need to experiment with new seasonings that please your palate (e.g., salt, spices, pepper, sauces).

CONSTIPATION

Constipation is not uncommon for patients taking TMZ and other chemotherapies. A fiber-rich diet, adequate hydration, and physical activity can help to minimize constipation, but when those measures aren't enough, stool softeners and laxatives may be required. Remember to discuss this problem with your provider, and notify him or her if you have not had a bowel movement in over 3 days. If you experience nausea/vomiting, or abdominal pain along with constipation, call your provider immediately because these symptoms may be a sign of a bowel obstruction.

FATIGUE

Feeling exhausted or extremely tired is probably the most common side effect that patients report. Many things can cause fatigue. Recent surgery and anesthesia combined with the body's healing process add to the fatigue, and it could take weeks to months to fully recover. Immediately adding radiation and chemotherapy after surgery can compound the fatigue and be overwhelming the first month or two afterward. Fatigue from radiation usually begins several weeks into treatment and can last several months.

Medical issues can also play a role in fatigue, including anemia and electrolyte imbalances caused by nausea, vomiting, and diarrhea.

Poor sleep can add to fatigue, so speak with your physician if you suffer from insomnia. Your physician may be able to prescribe something to help you get better rest. Stress, anxiety, and trying to maintain a family and employment can also add to fatigue.

No matter what the cause, you should discuss fatigue with your provider to help define and minimize it. The goal is to conserve your energy so that you can focus on doing the things most important to you. Tips to help you feel your best are as follows:

- Try to establish a routine.

- Listen to your body! Rest frequently.

- Mild exercise and activity such as a short walk will help to decrease fatigue.

- Make a list of things you need to accomplish and reach out to family and friends to help.

- Plan your activities at times of the day when you notice your energy levels are better.

BLOOD CLOTS

Although not exactly a side effect, brain tumor patients in general have a higher incidence of developing blood clots. The exact cause is still unknown. High-grade malignant glioma patients have an approximately 40% risk of developing clots at some time in their disease journey. These clots are called deep vein thromboses (DVTs) and usually occur in the veins of the leg. In some cases, a small piece may break off and travel through the bloodstream, which is called a thromboembolus. If these pieces travel and reach the lung (pulmonary embolus, or PE), they can cause severe breathing difficulty and even sudden death. Therefore, it is important that all brain cancer patients know the signs to look for as well as ways to help prevent developing clots. Although blood clots can occur without any symptoms at all, be sure to notify your provider immediately if you experience pain, swelling, or discoloration of your legs. He or she may order a Doppler ultrasound. which is a special test that looks at the blood flow in your legs' blood vessels. If you experience chest pain, chest pressure, or shortness of breath, you will need to be seen immediately in an emergency room. If you are diagnosed with a DVT or PE, you will be placed on blood thinners, or anticoagulants. Sometimes, filters (Greenfield filters) are placed in your inferior vena cava, which is the large vein in your abdomen that returns blood from your lower extremities to your heart and lungs. This filter will prevent blood clots in your legs from traveling anywhere else in your body.

FERTILITY

Many of the treatments used for brain tumors may affect a person's fertility, either temporarily or permanently. Speak to your medical treatment team for more information about how a specific treatment(s) may affect fertility. Many options are available to people whose treatment may affect their fertility. Before treatment begins, options such as sperm banking or egg or tissue freezing may be available. If these options are of interest, it is important to start investigating and making arrangements right away, as it may require weeks to set up and it should be done before treatment begins. Insurance coverage for these procedures varies widely, so it is also important to speak with your insurance company to find out what is covered.

After treatment, other options exist to pursue parenthood. For more information about fertility options before, during, and after treatment, see the comprehensive Web site, http://www.fertilehope.org.

SEXUALITY

Both brain tumors and the treatments for brain tumors may affect a person's sexuality. The reasons are different for each person and usually have both physiological and psychological components. Changes in sexuality may result from a decreased libido related to self-image as a person's body changes—scars, hair loss, weight changes—or they may result from side effects of the treatment such as fatigue. Most people do not feel comfortable discussing this problem with their doctor, although it might be important to them. The American Cancer Society offers booklets on its Web site (http://www.cancer.org) that are excellent sources of information.

Speak with a member of your healthcare team if you are having difficulty with sexual function.

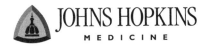

CHAPTER 5

STRAIGHT TALK—COMMUNICATION WITH FAMILY, FRIENDS, AND COWORKERS

Feelings of shock, confusion, and fear undoubtedly surrounded you when you were diagnosed with brain cancer. Your loved ones and friends, too, will experience these emotions. These feeling are all normal. Whom, when, and how much you tell depends largely on how much your diagnosis will impact them and how comfortable you are discussing your diagnosis. Many people understandably find it difficult to discuss their illness with others. First decide whom you need—and want—to tell. Those may be two different groups of people. People you need to tell are those who will be directly affected, including family members, your children, close friends, your boss, or others who live with you. These people will need to be aware that something very stressful is happening that may change their routines as well as have an emotional impact on them.

There are specialists, such as social workers or child-life specialists, who can help you talk about having cancer with children or others. Ask your doctor or nurse if these specialists are available where you are being treated. It is normal to want to protect your loved ones and friends, but doing so expends valuable energy that could be used to focus on getting well and fighting your cancer. Keeping your loved ones informed about how you feel, both physically and emotionally, will help them to better understand your challenges and therefore better equip them to provide support.

SHARING YOUR CANCER DIAGNOSIS

You will most likely have many different feelings and emotions as you learn more about your diagnosis and begin to make treatment decisions. The first step is to admit to yourself how you feel. Only you can decide when it is time to discuss your cancer with family and friends. Most individuals want and need to talk to someone. Telling those close to you can be difficult and can begin to make it all feel very real. Others may find that talking begins to allow them to solve problems, including other, nonmedical issues that need to be sorted out.

You should give some thought to how much about your brain cancer diagnosis you want to share. There is a lot to tell, including the type of cancer you have, treatments you may need, and the prognosis associated with brain cancer. You may find it helpful to start by making a list of people you will need to tell in person. People are often sobered by the news that someone has cancer. You may want to reassure them that you will do whatever is necessary to fight the cancer and would like to have their support and encouragement.

Think about which topics are too sensitive for you to discuss yet, and plan a response that is acceptable to you for when people ask you about these topics. Once you have shared what you wish to share, be prepared to change or end the conversation.

DEALING WITH UNEXPECTED FEELINGS

Even in the most loving families, members occasionally feel resentment when a family member becomes ill and cannot maintain his or her responsibilities for a while. This is especially true when the situation lasts for a long time. Whether they do so openly or not, family members may express anger toward you because their lives too are suddenly disrupted. While you may be the only available target for such anger, keep in mind that the situation, and not you, is at fault.

Though this kind of anger can be confusing and frustrating for everyone, it is a common response to a major life change. Sometimes you and your loved ones may feel out of step with each other. This can be upsetting, but remember, people react differently to stressful situations. People's experiences and personalities affect how they will react. Some loved ones may become absorbed in work, some may become overly involved in your treatment or personal life, and others may engage in activities outside the home and appear to not want to be involved at all. The best thing you can do for each other is be honest about what you are feeling. Fears about the future and feelings of guilt, resentment, and anger are often less frightening when you share them with others. Doing so can help all of you in the healing and acceptance process.

DISCUSSING YOUR FEARS

Most individuals after hearing your news will be curious about the next steps. They may want to know if you will need any additional surgery or if you will be undergoing radiation or chemotherapy. Answer their questions as best you can, but keep in mind that "I don't know" or "I'm not ready to think about that yet," are also good answers.

Generally, discussing your fears or concerns can put them into perspective. You may only realize your own true feelings when someone else asks a question. Once your fears and those of your loved ones are out in the open, they can stop growing and causing more misconceptions. Although it may be hard to do, discussing how you and your loved one are both coping with your diagnosis will make it easier to work together and make plans for the future.

TALKING WITH YOUR CHILDREN

If your children are young, don't assume they don't know that something significant has happened. Cancer, however, is often an unfamiliar concept to them. Do not overwhelm them with too much information. They tend to understand concrete ideas and make broad generalizations. How they react to upsetting news depends a lot on how the adults are handling it. Although youngsters will not understand what cancer is, they will understand what a boo-boo is; you can tell them that you have a boo-boo that the doctor needs to fix and that sometimes you feel sad about it and sometimes you are okay. As parents, we want to protect our children from fears, frustrations, and worries. Be careful, however, if children are not given honest explanations of the situation; they are likely to draw inaccurate, distressing conclusions as their imagination fills the gap. Try to maintain their routine as much as possible.

Depending on the age and maturity level of your child, you may want to consider attending a support/education group geared for children. It may be helpful for them to feel like they are not alone and that others have experienced what they are going through. Some hospitals even offer specialized education programs for children to introduce them to the hospital and discuss treatments that their parents may be going through. If possible, attend these programs with your child to help reduce his or her fears and anxiety. In addition, there are professionals such as social workers and child-life specialists who deal with these sorts of issues. Ask your doctor if these specialists are available at your treatment center.

Some treatments you may undergo can alter physical appearance (e.g., hair loss, facial swelling). It is important to prepare your child for such changes so he or she is not scared if they do, in fact, occur.

TALKING WITH TEENS

Teenagers may be anxious about how your cancer diagnosis will impact them. Will they get brain cancer some day too? How will their daily routines be affected? Sometimes teens can be resentful when asked to help out. You just need to understand where they are coming from. You will have to decide who will tell your teens and when, as well as how much detail and at what interval. Their knowledge base of cancer in general may be to associate it with death. Ask them what they know about cancer, and educate and inform them at their level. Reassure them to the appropriate degree, and be honest about your diagnosis and prognosis. Remember that teens still need to be teens. Tell them that you may need them to help out with tasks at home for a while, but also let them know that you do not want your treatment to totally disrupt their lives. The family as a whole will need to seek balance of responsibility.

TELLING PARENTS AND SIBLINGS

Telling your parents is also difficult. Parents often wish they could trade places and that they were the ones diagnosed, not you. They are used to making everything better for their children and may want to try to control the situation for you. They will become frustrated when they cannot control your treatment and recovery. They will need to be given constructive ways to help you—even if you don't think you need it at this time.

Siblings may fear that they will be the next to be diagnosed in the family. They may need support and information to help them cope with their own anxiety about your diagnosis of brain cancer. Reassure them that brain cancer is not hereditary or familial. Have them assist with information gathering and engage them in your treatment. Empower them with information that will help both of you. Family can be critical for providing and coordinating assistance during your treatment. Be sure to keep your family members informed of how you are doing and how treatment is progressing. Rely on their support.

DECIDING WHAT TO TELL YOUR BOSS AND COWORKERS

This decision is difficult. Whether or not to inform your coworkers about your illness is personal. Some people are open about their illnesses; others do not disclose anything. There are advantages to letting key people know because you will more than likely require some time off for treatment. You may choose to tell only your supervisor or closest associates, or you may decide to be public about your situation.

It is common to be concerned about maintaining your job after treatment. Fortunately, the American Disabilities Act provides some job protection. Providing that your cognition and mental abilities are adequate, and that you have not developed a seizure disorder that cannot be well controlled, you should be able to work with your boss on a schedule that will meet your medical needs as well as the needs of the employer. You are not actually required to tell your supervisor that you have cancer. It is fine to explain that you are under a doctor's care that will require you to miss time from work. Most people, however, will tell their boss that they have been diagnosed with cancer and will be undergoing whatever treatments have been recommended. You are not responsible for providing information about your prognosis.

As with friends and family, deciding what to tell coworkers can be difficult. Many will choose to inform coworkers in vague terms rather than provide them with the full details. This is your personal business so do what feels right and is the best in your situation. Offers of assistance from friends and coworkers are usually genuine. Their help and support may be very beneficial to you, so let them.

INFORMING YOUR FRIENDS

The decision to discuss your diagnosis with friends is yours alone. However, it is usually best to be honest about your cancer with people close to you. Keeping it a secret could cause you more stress at a time when you could use the support of others. Often, people feel awkward and uncomfortable. Some may even avoid talking to you after they hear the news. It isn't that they don't care; more likely, they don't know what to say, at least without being emotional at the same time. They may be frightened about the possibility of losing you. They may feel that it is better to say nothing than risk saying the wrong thing. Some may withdraw themselves, and others may become overly considerate or intrusive. Let them know that even though the diagnosis is upsetting to hear, you need their support. Most likely, your friends and family will want to help you, so let them. Be specific as to what you want them to do; this makes it easier for everyone.

KEEPING FRIENDS AND FAMILY UPDATED

During and after treatment, keeping people updated on your situation can be a job in itself. Some individuals find it helpful to assign this task to someone who can serve as the "information center." He or she will provide updates on how you are doing, what treatments you are currently undergoing, test results, and so on. There are a number of online resources for posting such information, and many of them are free. These Web sites can be personalized and will keep all of your friends and family informed. Some sites include a patient care journal, a photo gallery, and even a guest book where visitors can post messages of support and encouragement. If a formal Web site is more than you are looking for, simple emails are another excellent way to ensure that all of your loved ones are informed without having to call each one. Enlist the help of someone to gather all important email addresses, and send out broadcast emails to everyone at once with periodic updates. You will find that these options are huge time savers, reduce the burden to you, and ensure the accuracy and consistency of the information being provided.

RECRUITING SUPPORT FROM FAMILY AND FRIENDS

People will undoubtedly ask what they can do to help you. It may be helpful to identify a coordinator early on who can delegate tasks to your support team. Among the many things people can do are to help drive you to your appointments, drive your children to school and events, run errands, make meals (that can be put in the freezer), babysit, help with the housework, or add you to a prayer list at church. Remember that these people want to do something to help and would not offer if they did not sincerely want to provide you with that assistance. Support from others is an important part of your treatment plan for you and for your family.

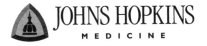

CHAPTER 6

MAINTAINING BALANCE—WORK AND LIFE DURING TREATMENT

PLANNING YOUR CARE AND MINIMIZING DISRUPTIONS IN YOUR LIFE

The last thing you expected to be was the person in your family needing help! You are used to being the one in control, taking care of the family and home, not the one needing care. You are accustomed to juggling busy schedules, functioning as a spouse, parent, babysitter, nurse, financial manager, bread winner, counselor, chauffeur, and magician in the family most of the time. For this reason, you might not be good at asking for and accepting help from others. Your brain cancer treatment may alter roles, play havoc with schedules, and create additional stress, including financial concerns for you, family members, and friends helping during this time. It is inevitable, but it can be managed.

MONEY

A brain cancer diagnosis may require cutting back or even discontinuing work completely either temporarily or permanently. Decreased employment can reduce the amount of money that your family has to spend or save. If you are unable to work, someone else in your family may need to get a job to help make ends meet. You will also have to learn about the benefits provided by your health insurance company so you will be prepared for what tests, procedures, services, and medications are covered.

LIVING ARRANGEMENTS

Sometimes, especially if you live alone, having brain cancer may require that you move in with someone, either a friend or a family member, so you can get the care and help you need. This can be hard because you may feel like you are losing your independence. If you do have to be away from home for care and treatment, be sure to take a few personal effects with you to help make your stay comfortable and as pleasant as possible.

PREPARING FOR SURGERY

Before your surgery, make sure that you have a basic understanding about the procedure that will be performed and what recovery will be like. Keep in mind that the recovery period will vary and depend upon your age and tolerance, and what procedure is performed. For more information about surgical preparation, please refer back to Chapter 3.

PREPARING FOR RADIATION

Consider scheduling your treatment appointments at the beginning or end of the day rather than in the middle if possible. Radiation treatment is daily and you will want to cause as little disruption to your daily routines as possible. Most radiation facilities have patients in and out in 30 to 60 minutes. The actual treatment itself lasts only minutes.

If you are also taking TMZ during your initial radiation, remember that it should be taken on an empty stomach with a full glass of water about 1 hour before your radiation treatment is scheduled. Medications to prevent nausea and vomiting can also be taken at this time.

PREPARING FOR CHEMOTHERAPY

If you are scheduled to have systemic therapy, make a chart of when your treatments will be, which day you will see your doctor, and when you will need to have your blood drawn. If possible, having treatments toward the end of the week will allow you to have the weekend to recoup and hopefully provide the extra help you may need. You will need someone to drive you to your appointment and take you home afterward for at least your first cycle of treatment. This is because you don't know how you will feel afterward, and often premedications are given that may make you drowsy. You may be in the infusion center several hours receiving your chemotherapy, so plan accordingly.

Hair loss is a potential side effect of both radiation and some chemotherapy agents. You may want to consider cutting your hair short prior to it falling out. Friends and family can supply you with various head coverings—baseball caps, turbans, hats, etc.

PREVENTING INFECTION AND STAYING HEALTHY DURING TREATMENT

Systemic chemotherapy may cause your white blood cell count to decrease. Depending on the specific agent, it is often possible to forecast when your blood counts may drop but it may happen at any time. It is especially important during the time when your white blood cell count is less than adequate to be careful and protect yourself because you are particularly vulnerable to getting a cold, flu, or other forms of infection during this time. You will want to be particularly careful and avoid contact with children, who are often contagious but do not appear ill. Wearing a mask while in closed environments, and frequent hand washing with soap or hand sanitizers can be very beneficial in helping you prevent infections. Try to maintain a balanced diet; one that is rich in washed fruits and vegetables can help to improve your immune system and resistance.

Depending on the time of year you are receiving treatment, getting a flu shot is highly recommended. In some cases, your physician may recommend getting one flu shot early in the season and then repeating one later just to help maintain your defense.

CONTINUING WORK AND RETURNING TO WORK

If and when you return to work is a personal and difficult decision. You have to be ready. Even after surgery, your treatment course is at an early stage. You will initially have daily appointments for approximately 6 weeks while receiving radiation and concurrent chemotherapy. Most patients find maintaining employment during this phase of treatment extremely difficult to manage. Once this stage of treatment is completed, your visits will change to office visits and lab appointments several times per month. You will have to see how you feel at this time before deciding about your return to work. The decision about if and when to return to work is made in consultation with your physician.

Some people, if mentally and physically capable, find that returning to work at least part-time allows them to get back to their normal life. It may also help to motivate them and distract them from thinking about their cancer diagnosis. You may find that your workplace is a supportive environment. Most employers will try to work with you while you are in treatment. Still it is a good idea to keep careful records of all your discussions with your employer or benefits office. There are federal regulations that protect your rights while in treatment—namely, the American Disabilities Act. Legal assistance is available to you if you feel you have been treated unfairly at your place of employment.

Many companies have a medical leave of absence program or disability leave. Depending on your employer, you may or may not receive wages during this period. The best part about these plans is that they continue your health insurance while you are absent from your job. Telecommuting is also an option that allows you the freedom to work around your treatment schedule. If your job can be completed in your home office, you may want to suggest this to your employer. If you are considering cutting back your hours to part-time, remember this may affect your benefits as well. Be sure to discuss all of your questions and concerns with your employer's benefits office before finalizing your decision.

If you decide to return, there may be times when you will need to arrive late or leave early to keep your appointments or receive treatment. Try to inform your employer and your coworkers as soon as possible so it will be easier for you and prevent disruptions in your work as well as allow time to find coverage for your missed time.

FINDING MORE TIME AND MODIFYING YOUR PRIORITIES

Most people find it hard to fit everything into their family schedule even without the demands of a new cancer diagnosis and treatment. Consider the following tips for finding more time for yourself and your family:

- Take advantage of free and low-cost delivery services. Many stores offer online shopping and home delivery. Many items can be delivered to your home, including groceries, prescriptions, DVDs, stamps, and even dry cleaning.

- Spend less time in the kitchen. Make double recipes and freeze half for a later dinner, or purchase nutritious prepared meals and frozen foods available at your grocery store. Simple meals, such as sandwiches or scrambled eggs, can substitute for a more elaborate meal.

- Do not try to clean the whole house. Concentrate on what matters to you, like having the dishes or laundry done. If possible, hire a cleaning service or even a neighborhood kid to help you clean.

- Reconsider your family schedule. If your spouse or loved ones are involved in many activities, ask them to pick two or three and take a break from others.

- Rearrange your own activities and focus on one or two that are really important to you. Do not commit to any new activities until you know you are up to it and have time for them.

Cancer and cancer treatment are tough on a physical and emotional level. With all the demands on your time, it can be easy to forget to take time for yourself. Decide which tasks are priorities for you and which tasks you can ask someone else to do or just leave undone. Setting aside time to do something you enjoy or just to relax and rest is an important part of the healing process. Ultimately, when you take care of yourself, you will have more energy and patience needed to fight your disease and juggle all of your familial responsibilities.

Remember, there are people who can help you with planning and coping with the changes in your life. Don't be afraid to ask for help from the many professionals available to you, such as a social worker, chaplain, or counselor, if the road gets bumpy. Your doctor or nurse can help you make the initial contact.

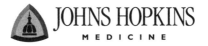

CHAPTER 7

SURVIVING BRAIN CANCER—
RE-ENGAGING IN MIND AND BODY
HEALTH AFTER TREATMENT

SURVIVORSHIP

When are you a cancer survivor? Some people consider themselves survivors the minute they are diagnosed and start treatment. Others don't consider themselves survivors until they have completed their treatment. In general, survivorship is so much more than a definition. It relates to your mental and physical well-being after diagnosis.

Once treatment stops, cancer survivors find themselves entering a whole new world—one filled with many new questions. Completing your prescribed treatment is surely a time to rejoice. You are probably relieved and happy to put the experience behind you; yet at the same time, you may feel sad and worried. You have been focused on actively fighting your disease, and now that your treatment is completed, you may feel a letdown and fear that your cancer will return. Maybe you feel as if you haven't done enough or as if there should be something you can do to stop your cancer from recurring. All of these feelings are normal.

When treatment ends, you may expect life to return to the way it was before you were diagnosed with brain cancer, but it can take time for you to recover. You may have permanent scars or hair loss and may not be able to do some of the things you were once able to do easily. You may think that others see you differently now, or you may view yourself in a different way. One of the hardest realities after treatment is not knowing what happens next. Those who have gone through cancer treatment often describe the first several months as a time of change. It is not so much "getting back to normal" as finding out what is "normal" for you now. People often say their life has new meaning, or they look at things differently. They realize they may need to shift their priorities to enjoy life. You should also focus on maintaining a healthy lifestyle, eating well, exercising, and spending more time doing things that bring happiness to yourself or others.

Unfortunately, some people allow the cancer to consume their lives, even if their disease is currently stable without signs of recurrence. They may feel upset with themselves, their doctors, their family, or even their religion for letting them down. Some patients become so involved in their cancer care that when they are done, they actually feel lost and do not know what to do next. They are constantly thinking about the disease recurring and allow those thoughts to interfere with many of their daily activities, such as sleeping or eating. Though these patients are living, they are not surviving. Of course, it is common for every patient to have these feelings or thoughts at some time, but it is important to prevent them from taking over every moment. Remember, most cancer centers offer support for cancer survivors, their spouses, and families. Participating in a support group may help you to maintain or regain balance in your life.

COUNSELING

Many people experience a feeling of fatigue or general weakness after their cancer treatment, sometimes affecting their activity levels. If you feel you are having a hard time adjusting, you may consider seeking help. Your doctor or nurse can help refer you to a counselor. Don't feel like you have failed getting yourself back on track. This readjustment process is very hard. Many people can benefit from seeing a therapist to help them re-engage in their lives physically and emotionally. Sometimes we need a professional sounding board to hear our hidden thoughts and fears, which can help us to gain perspective about what and what not to spend our energy worrying about. There is no operator's manual for this task, so consider taking assistance from someone who is professionally trained if you are having difficulty.

MANAGING SIDE EFFECTS

In Chapter 4, we discussed some of the more common side effects associated with your diagnosis and treatment. Unfortunately, it is not uncommon for some of these side effects to linger for months or even years after your treatment. You may be dealing with residual side effects such as headaches, motor and sensory loss, fatigue, and difficulty with memory, speech, or cognition, as well as other difficulties. Don't expect to feel back to yourself right away. There is a time of psychological and physical adjustment. Your body and brain need time to heal. Allow them time to recover. (See Chapter 4 for the management of side effects.)

LIVING A HEALTHIER LIFESTYLE

Now that you are a cancer survivor, it is important that you take charge of your overall health. Doing so will not only make you stronger, but it may improve your emotional health as well. There are many ways to accomplish this. A few suggestions follow.

NUTRITION

Everyone should be mindful of their eating habits. However, now that you have been diagnosed with brain cancer, nutrition is even more important. Eating a well-balanced diet, maintaining a healthy weight, and exercising will help you to feel better about yourself and life as a whole. Your immune system will be boosted, you will sleep better, and you will feel stronger.

WEIGHT

Along with a healthy diet comes the ability to maintain a healthy weight. Weight management is especially difficult for brain cancer patients because of the frequent use of steroids (Decadron) to control brain swelling. Steroids increase appetite and cause the redistribution of fat cells. There is not much you can do to stop these side effects. However, you can minimize them by making better choices about satisfying your hunger. For instance, try to eat lots of fresh fruits and vegetables as an alternative to cookies, pastries, or snack foods that for the most part contain empty calories. The less weight you gain, the easier it will be to remain active and ambulatory.

EXERCISE

As mentioned earlier, exercise is an important part of healthy living. Consult your physician to choose an exercise program that is right for you. A nice walk for a half hour three to five times a week is a good start. Start slowly and work up to a good pace. If you are able, add some strength training with 3- to 5-pound weights. Not only will doing so help to maintain/increase muscle strength (which also can be adversely affected with steroid use), but it will help to keep your bones strong. Staying active can also help prevent blood clots in your legs, which are known to occur in patients with brain cancer.

AVOIDING BAD HABITS

Along with your healthy diet and exercise regimen, try to avoid dangerous habits. If you smoke, quit, and avoid second-hand smoke. Encourage friends and family to quit smoking or refrain from smoking when they are around you. Minimize your alcohol intake too. If you choose to drink, limit yourself to one drink a day. Be sure to talk with your physician, especially if you are on seizure medication, before drinking any alcoholic beverages.

AVOIDING STRESS

No matter where you are in the process of treating your brain cancer—just starting, in the middle, or at the end—you will encounter stress. The stress may be related to your cancer and cancer care or to the daily stressors of life, including family, financial issues, etc. Stress can not only detract from overall physical and emotional well-being, it can also weaken your immune system. Your immune system plays a critical role in fighting your cancer as well as infection.

Not much can be done to avoid certain stressors, but how you cope with and respond to them is important. Some patients learn meditation or other relaxation techniques. Most importantly, learn to let the little things go, thereby allowing you to focus on life's more important issues. Keep things in perspective. Remember, you are a cancer survivor.

MEMORY AND COGNITIVE CHANGES

As discussed in Chapter 4, brain tumor patients have difficulty with cognition for a number of reasons. The already troublesome effects of a brain tumor are exacerbated first by surgery and medications, then by radiation, then by chemotherapy—all in a short time. Mental functioning is understandably affected. Refer to the list on pages 68–69 for techniques that can help to heighten memory and concentration.

SETTING NEW GOALS

You have just completed treatment that has likely affected many facets of your life. This is an ideal time to step back and reassess your life. Issues will arise that include whether you are able to continue working, and if so, whether you will work full- or part-time. You must also consider how you want to spend time with your family and friends. Will you try a new hobby, something you have always wanted to do? Is this the time to change and devote more attention to living a healthier lifestyle?

Whatever you decide, this is the time to set short-term goals. Some reach out to support groups as a source of education and support; others find keeping a journal beneficial. Most importantly, keep communication lines open. Your family and friends may expect things to return to how they were before your diagnosis. This may not be possible and may require adjustment on everyone's part. Share your goals with those around you, and help them to understand and support you in the process of reaching these goals.

FAITH, RELIGION, OR SPIRITUALITY

Being diagnosed with cancer can undoubtedly affect your spiritual outlook. After you have completed each phase of treatment, you and your loved ones may struggle to understand why you had to endure such a trial in your life. Some individuals' spirituality may grow even stronger and more vital; others may find themselves questioning their faith and wondering about the meaning of life and their purpose in it.

Through faith, many cancer survivors are able to find new meaning in their lives and help make sense of their cancer. Religion can also provide an outlet for coping and recovering from cancer. Seeking answers and searching for personal meaning in spirituality can offer hope, perspective, and comfort.

SEEING THE WORLD THROUGH DIFFERENT EYES

Your brain cancer diagnosis has likely changed your life and deeply affected those closest to you. You may have a new perspective on things and realize how precious life is. This is the time for you not only to focus on yourself and your own health, but that of your family and friends as well. You may want to get involved in a support group so you can share your experience with other brain cancer survivors and help individuals who are just starting their journey with this disease. Let your doctor know you would be willing to speak with another person who is facing surgery, radiation, or systemic therapy for brain cancer. You may also want to consider getting involved by volunteering for a brain cancer organization to help raise awareness and funding for efforts to find a cure. Make sure you are far enough along in your recovery as not to jeopardize your own health. Helping others can be very rewarding and is a great way to give back as well as help yourself.

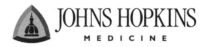

CHAPTER 8

MANAGING RISK—WHAT IF MY CANCER COMES BACK?

T he risk of recurrence remains one of the most feared issues that people deal with when they are diagnosed with brain cancer, particularly after they have finished their initial treatment. Recurrence for a patient diagnosed with a high-grade malignant glioma is almost certain. The goal of treatment is to prevent recurrence for as long as possible and, if it does recur, to enact a treatment regimen best suited for the individual's needs. Is more surgery an option? Are there other chemotherapies or treatments that can slow the growth of the tumor? What about clinical trials? Is more radiation a possibility?

MONITORING FOR RECURRENCE

MRIs are the standard neuroradiological study for assessing brain tumor status. After your initial surgery is performed, a new MRI, usually obtained before you are discharged from the hospital to determine the extent of tumor removal/resection, will serve as your new radiographic baseline. This MRI scan will also be used to plan your radiation treatment.

Generally, the next scheduled MRI scan is done a month or two after your radiation treatment is completed. This scan can often be somewhat difficult to interpret due to all the recent surgery and treatment, which can mimic radiographic progression. Within the first 3 months after completion of radiation treatment and concomitant (at the same time) TMZ administration, diagnosis of recurrence can be indistinguishable from pseudoprogression on the MRI scan. If clinically you are doing well, it is not uncommon to repeat another MRI in 4 to 8 weeks. Stabilization or improvement in the radiological picture should occur within 3 months from the end of radiation treatment if the findings are pseudoprogression. Conversely, true progression will not radiographically improve.

Thereafter, an MRI is done about every 2 months or 2 cycles of TMZ. After your systemic chemotherapy regimen with TMZ has been completed, MRI scans are generally recommended every 2 to 4 months. If 2 years have elapsed with no radiographic evidence of recurrence, then decreasing MRI scan frequency may be considered.

You will receive MRI scans to assess tumor activity for the rest of your life. If your brain tumor shows radiographic evidence of progression/recurrence and is not responding to the current treatment, the TMZ or other systemic treatment will be stopped and a new treatment strategy will be discussed by your doctor.

TREATMENT OPTIONS

As with the guidelines for newly diagnosed patients listed on pages 30–31, the NCCN offers treatment guidelines for patients with recurrent high-grade gliomas. They are summarized in Table 2.

There is no magic involved in choosing your treatment regimen and no absolutes in determining what to do next. The NCCN guidelines are well established and respected but are just guidelines that physicians use for treating. At every juncture, a thoughtful discussion between you and your physician should take place. This discussion should take into account your wishes, the specifics of your disease, your tumor's location and size, your tumor's operability, your overall state of health, your body's likely ability to tolerate prospective treatments, and your response to past treatments.

MORE SURGERY

There is general consensus that if your brain cancer has recurred in an area that is amenable to surgery, then this is the first and most viable option. Several benefits can be obtained by this option.

First, you will be able to get confirmation from the pathologist of what exactly is responsible for the radiological changes. Is it tumor recurrence or could it be what is commonly known as "treatment effect"? Treatments—radiation and/or chemotherapy—sometimes produce radiological (MRI) and clinical changes that suggest tumor regrowth. In such cases, the pathologist's microscopic examination may reveal a few tumor cells, but the changes can be attributed to treatment, not to tumor regrowth. If the pathology reveals only treatment effect, it is unlikely that you will require any

Table 2 Standard Guideline for Treatment of Recurrent Anaplastic Gliomas/Glioblastomas

RADIOGRAPHIC RESULTS	RECURRENCE	SURGICAL OPTIONS	LOCAL THERAPY	TREATMENT	NO TREATMENT
Follow up imaging (MRI/CT) reveals recurrent or progressive disease for anaplastic gliomas and glioblastoma *including mixed anaplastic oligoastrocytoma (AOA), anaplastic astrocytoma (AA), anaplastic oligodendroglioma (AO), gliosarcoma and other rare anaplastic gliomas **Consider MR spectroscopy, MR perfusion, or brain PET scan to assist in distinguishing active tumor from radiation necrosis or treatment effect.	Diffuse or in more than one area of the brain	Usually not indicated unless for palliative symptomatic management of a large lesion	Not indicated	Best supportive care if performance status (KPS) is poor or Systemic chemotherapy or Surgery for symptomatic large lesions	Best supportive care only
	Recurrence from within or surrounding the original tumor cavity	Resectable/removable	Resection with carmustine (BCNU) chemotherapy wafers	Best supportive care if performance status (KPS) is poor or Systemic chemotherapy or Consider re-irradiation (*especially if long interval since prior RT and/or if there was a good response to prior RT)	
		Unresectable	Resection without carmustine (BCNU) chemotherapy wafers		

additional treatment to stop your tumor from growing at that time because it has been established that there is currently no activity.

Second, if there is active tumor recurrence, by removing as much tumor as possible, you receive the benefit of decreasing "tumor burden," or the amount of residual tumor cells left behind. Decreasing tumor burden minimizes the work that the next treatment or systemic chemotherapy has to do.

Lastly, but of equal importance, often a tumor-reductive surgery may help to improve or even alleviate symptoms that are caused by mass effect of the tumor pressing on functional surrounding brain tissues. Swelling may decrease, and therefore your need for steroids may be reduced. Local therapy with the BCNU polymer wafers (Gliadel wafers) should be considered at this time unless contraindicated by tumor location. You may have the BCNU wafers implanted more than once. Be sure to discuss with your surgeon whether you are a candidate.

There is no limit to how many surgeries you can have to remove brain cancer, although each subsequent surgical procedure may have slightly more associated risks than the one prior. These risks are especially important when considering your body's ability to heal and prevent infection. Subsequent craniotomies, especially after recent irradiation and chemotherapy, may present problems with incisional healing, breakdown, and infection. Surgeons will usually offer and agree to more surgery if you are in good enough condition to tolerate the procedure and anesthesia, but more importantly if they feel you will receive benefit from the surgery. Be sure to discuss the risks and potential benefits with your surgeon before considering a trip back to the operating room.

TEMOZOLOMIDE

Many neuro-oncologists feel that restarting TMZ may provide benefit to their patients if they have had a favorable response to the concomitant/adjuvant dosing of TMZ—if, for example, they completed radiation with TMZ and then completed the six cycles of postradiation or adjuvant TMZ with reasonable tolerance. Tolerance means there were no prolonged or life-threatening hematologic (blood count) side effects and the treatment regimen was completed without disease progression. The patient's disease must then be stable for at least 6 months after the discontinuance of TMZ. It is then often considered reasonable by the neuro-oncology community to restart TMZ as a systemic chemotherapy. In short, if your brain cancer had clear response noted by its lack of progression during the previous treatment, it may be felt that you have a significant chance to respond again.

BCNU

BCNU is an anticancer chemotherapy drug and is classified as an "alkylating agent." BCNU is used to treat various primary brain tumors, including glioblastoma multiforme, brain stem glioma, astrocytomas, and others, as well as some metastatic brain tumors. Other cancers treated with BCNU are multiple myeloma, Hodgkin disease, non-Hodgkin lymphomas, melanoma, lung cancer, and colon cancer.

Administration of BCNU

BCNU is given intravenously (IV) every 6 weeks. The amount of BCNU given is based on a calculation of your height and weight as well as other factors such as your general health. It is generally dosed 150–200 mg/m^2 and is given every 6 weeks over 2 hours. Nausea and vomiting after IV administration of BCNU are noted frequently. This toxicity appears within 2 hours of dosing, usually lasting 4 to 6 hours. Prior administration of antiemetics is effective in diminishing and sometimes preventing gastrointestinal distress.

Side Effects of BCNU

People receiving BCNU may experience a variety of related side effects. These effects are dose dependent and are most severe with higher dosages. The side effects include but are not limited to:

- *Nausea and vomiting.* These effects usually begin within 2 to 4 hours of the infusion and last for about 4 to 6 hours.

- *Facial flushing.*

- *Pain and burning at the injection sight.*

- *Low blood counts.* BCNU may affect white blood cells and platelets, which can put individuals at risk for infection and/or bleeding. Effects on blood counts are expected to begin 7 to 14 days after the infusion, may worsen at 3 to 5 weeks after an infusion, and may take up to 60 days to resolve.

AVASTIN

Avastin (bevacizumab) is the newest FDA-approved treatment for recurrent malignant gliomas. It was first approved for use in other types of cancers, including colorectal cancer, non-small cell lung cancer, and renal cell cancer. In the spring of 2009, Avastin gained FDA approval to treat a particular type of brain tumor—glioblastoma multiforme.

As a monoclonal antibody, Avastin is not considered chemotherapy but instead a biologic therapy. By blocking a protein called vascular endothelial growth factor, a key component in new blood vessel formation, Avastin attempts to inhibit new blood vessel growth to the tumor. If the tumor cannot make new blood vessels, it has a harder time growing. Halting this type of new blood vessel growth is called anti-angiogenesis. Avastin is an anti-angiogenesis agent. Avastin also helps to repair the blood–brain barrier, which helps to reduce brain swelling.

Administration of Avastin

Avastin is given intravenously every 2 weeks for treatment in gliomas. To avoid any possible infusion reactions, the drug is given over 90 minutes for the first infusion, followed by 60 minutes for the second infusion, and 30 minutes for all remaining infusions. There is no need to take antiemetics prior to receiving Avastin, as this drug does not cause nausea or vomiting, nor does it cause hair loss.

In many cases, Avastin is given in conjunction with another chemotherapy agent (either oral or intravenous). Several clinical trials are currently testing various combinations of therapies with Avastin in an effort to find the most effective combination or multiple effective combinations.

Side Effects of Avastin

Overall, Avastin is generally well tolerated. Expected and common side effects include high blood pressure, protein in the urine, delayed wound healing, fatigue, and mild nosebleeds.

There are a few rare but serious risks with Avastin, which occur in approximately 1%–4% of treatments. These risks include gastrointestinal perforation (anywhere along the gastrointestinal tract), severe bleeding, blood clots, stroke, heart failure, and kidney damage. If any of these serious events occur, Avastin therapy is stopped indefinitely.

CLINICAL TRIALS

As discussed in detail in Chapter 3, the goal of clinical trials is to find better ways to treat cancer and help people who have cancer. Many types of treatment are tested in this way, such as new drugs, new approaches to surgery or radiation therapy, new combinations of treatments, or new methods such as gene therapy, vaccination, immunotherapy, etc. Because it is unlikely for the therapies that are currently available to be curative once your brain cancer returns, you may be offered a clinical trial. Clinical trials can be a viable option for people with cancer. If the idea of a clinical trial appeals to you, then you may want to consider enrolling in one early in your disease process when it is most likely that you will meet the eligibility criteria. Many clinical trials set eligibility restrictions based on the amount and types of treatment patients have previously received. For example, a clinical trial may allow you to have had only one prior systemic chemotherapy. Therefore, if you have completed radiation and TMZ, you would be eligible, but if you decide to decline the trial for another systemic chemotherapy and then have another recurrence, you would no longer be eligible to receive treatment from that trial.

RE-IRRADIATION

For the most part, patients who have high-grade malignant gliomas are given a lifetime dose of radiation shortly after the initial diagnosis. In rare cases, when a significant time between initial irradiation and recurrence has occurred, a radiation oncologist may consider delivering additional radiation as a palliative effort. The total dose delivered, however, in re-irradiation for high-grade malignant gliomas is 30–35 cGy, or about half of the initial prescribed dose.

RADIOSURGERY/GAMMA KNIFE/CYBERKNIFE

There is no conclusive data to support the use of focused radiation in the treatment of gliomas. However, there are centers across the United States that do incorporate these treatments in the management of this disease. Gamma knife and radiosurgery are delivery systems for "focused radiation." These treatments are designed to treat tumors with very well-defined margins. By definition, gliomas have very ill-defined and infiltrative margins and are therefore not ideal candidates for these treatments. Although the Johns Hopkins Brain Cancer Center does not use this treatment in the management of high-grade gliomas, it is important for patients to be aware of and knowledgeable about the indications for focused radiation.

There are many treatment options for recurrent high-grade malignant gliomas. The NCCN has provided guidelines to assist practitioners in making the appropriate decisions. Deciding which treatment to receive when tumors recur requires a serious and comprehensive discussion with your physician. Be sure to discuss the potential risks and benefits of each option as well as the impact on your quality of life before you make your decision.

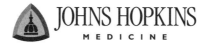

CHAPTER 9

MY CANCER ISN'T CURABLE—
WHAT NOW?

High-grade malignant gliomas (grade III anaplastic astrocytoma/oligodendroglioma and grade IV glioblastoma multiforme) are the most common and most aggressive type of primary brain cancer. Although they are the most prevalent form of primary brain cancer, they do not behave like many other systemic cancers in that recurrence or metastases outside of the brain are extremely rare. If and when gliomas recur, they usually do so within 2 cm of the original site. Thus, these tumors usually come back along the margins of the resection cavity or borders of the original tumor. Approximately 10%–20% of the time, high-grade malignant gliomas may develop new lesions at distant sites, in another lobe of the brain, or within the spinal column.

Metastases outside of the brain or CNS from high-grade malignant gliomas are rare, with a reported frequency of less than 0.5%, occurring in the lymph nodes, lungs, bone, and liver. Most of the reported cases associated with metastases outside the brain or spine occurred in patients who had previous surgery for placement of a ventriculoperitoneal shunt or stereotactic biopsy. Because the cases are so few, the causative mechanism that helps to enable metastases in these patients is not well understood.

Although metastases from high-grade malignant gliomas are rare, local recurrences can be extremely aggressive. As these tumors grow, it is not uncommon for them to encompass an entire lobe of the brain and even cross into the other hemisphere of the brain. As the brain cancer spreads, it often involves more functional areas of the brain. Patients may develop more and more neurologic deficits and symptoms. They may develop weakness in one or both sides of the body, have difficulty thinking and speaking clearly, or have problems hearing or seeing. Which symptoms individuals manifest depends entirely upon which direction the tumor cells grow and which functional brain tissue they destroy.

When treatments are no longer effective at stopping the progression of the cancer and recurrence becomes so extensive that neurologic function is destroyed, a shift from quantity of time to quality of life begins. When exactly to stop treating and fighting the disease is an individual decision. The timing of this decision is often very difficult. It is extremely important to discuss this ahead of time with your family. Be clear about your desires and wishes because there may come a time when your brain cancer will render you unable to make clear decisions for yourself.

PROGNOSIS

High-grade malignant gliomas cannot be cured. The prognosis for these patients is generally poor, especially for older patients. About half of all people diagnosed with malignant gliomas are alive 1 year after diagnosis, and 25% are after 2 years. If the diagnosis is an anaplastic astrocytoma, survival is generally estimated at about 3 years. Glioblastoma multiforme has a worse prognosis, with less than a 12-month average survival after diagnosis.

These numbers are frightening. Keep in mind that these statistics are based on all patients. There are many factors that affect prognosis and survival time, including the individual's age and neurologic function at diagnosis and after resection, extent of resection, preexisting medical conditions, tumor size, tumor location, and specific DNA alterations and pathologic characteristics, to name a few.

SETTING SHORT-TERM GOALS

It would be wonderful if we could all make plans for 10 years from now and expect to be here to fulfill them. Unfortunately, this may not be a realistic goal when dealing with brain cancer because it is incurable. Begin by setting short-term goals. First, see how well you recover from the surgery. Then reevaluate to determine how the cancer responds to radiation and chemotherapy.

There are people who have survived 5, 10, and even 15 years or longer after being diagnosed with brain cancer, but unfortunately just a few. Talk frankly with your treatment team so you are prepared and know what to expect. Ask your doctor to thoroughly explain the treatment plan including the schedule of when the imaging studies are going to be performed to evaluate the effectiveness of the treatments. Use these milestones to make your next set of short-term goals. Your time is limited, so it is better to use it wisely when you are still feeling well enough to enjoy it. Make a list of things you would like to accomplish in a timely manner. Discuss these goals with your loved ones and make plans to complete those that are possible.

QUANTITY OF LIFE VERSUS QUALITY OF LIFE

Regardless of your disease status, quality of life should always be at the forefront of your thoughts. This means that living to be 100 years old in constant pain, unable to care for your own daily needs and not enjoying being alive is by far less desirable than living a shorter life in which you feel well, enjoy your family, and are happy. There should always be an emphasis on not just quantity of life—staying alive—but quality of life, making sure you enjoy the days you are alive. Along with your short-term goals, try to decide where you want to be, what you want to do, and with whom you want to spend the time you have left.

Not all issues that affect quality of life are apparent to your treatment team. For instance, if you are in pain or are having headaches, let your physician know, as he or she may be able to adjust your medications to reduce the swelling that is causing your headaches or even prescribe you pain medication. Don't be afraid to make your providers aware of any and all symptoms; they may be able to reduce or eliminate them. It is up to you to find the balance between quality of life and quantity of life.

DECIDING TO STOP TREATMENT

Asking your doctor when to stop treatment is not easy, nor is it an easy question for him or her to answer. Still, having a candid discussion about stopping treatment is very valuable. As discussed earlier, you may want to have a discussion with your physician ahead of time, while you are still doing well and have all of your mental abilities intact. This may require that you meet one-on-one with your doctor when family is not with you. You may find it easier to have this discussion without your spouse, child, or parent sitting beside you because these loved ones won't want to hear the answers to some of the difficult questions. Make sure your wishes and desires are well understood by your provider, as he or she may need to assist your family in making the right decision at the right time on your behalf.

Treatment, in general, can continue as long as you are responding to it without severe side effects, there are treatment options to offer you, and your quality of life is acceptable to you. There may come a time when your doctor advises against continuing treatment for your cancer. This may be because you are too sick to tolerate any more treatment or because the treatment is no longer effective at controlling your brain cancer.

You will want your doctor to be honest with you and your family. Physicians are trained to make people better—to heal, cure, alleviate pain, and reduce suffering. Having to tell patients that continuing treatment will not benefit them is very hard. However, even though your doctor does not recommend any additional therapy or you decide to stop, you will still be taken care of. Your treatment team will still be actively involved in trying to maintain as much quality of life and control of your symptoms as possible.

Be sure to have your affairs in order and your wishes well known. There is a tendency to postpone these matters. Everyone, even those without cancer, should have their affairs in order. Life is unpredictable. Fatal car accidents happen. You are in a situation that is providing you a window into your future. Take advantage of this unusual knowledge by making sure your will and advance directives are in place, your finances are in order, and your wishes are well known to your next of kin.

PALLIATIVE AND HOSPICE CARE

Palliative and hospice care are approaches that focus on you and maintaining your quality of life—actively treating your physical symptoms as well as psychological and spiritual concerns, and ultimately assisting you and those closest to you with bereavement. The goals of palliative care are to help with personal care, symptom control, and maintenance of quality of life. You may often continue with treatment of your cancer while receiving this additional support.

Hospice care provides humane and compassionate care for people who are in the last phases of incurable diseases so they may live as fully and comfortably as possible. The goal of hospice is to enable patients to continue an alert, pain-free life and to manage other symptoms so their last days may be spent with dignity and quality, surrounded by their loved ones. Hospice treats the person and not the disease. It provides family-centered care and involves the patient and the family in decision making. Care is provided for the patient and the family 24 hours a day, 7 days a week. Hospice care can be given in your home, a hospital, a nursing home, or a private hospice facility. Most hospice care in the United States is given in the home, with family members serving as the main hands-on caregivers.

Hospice is suitable when you will no longer benefit from cancer treatment and you are expected to live 6 months or less. You, your family, and your doctor decide together when hospice care should begin. Because this decision can be so difficult, it is unfortunately often not started soon enough. Sometimes the doctor, patient, and/or family members resist the decision because they feel it sends a message of hopelessness. This is not true. If you get better or the disease goes into remission, you can be taken out of the hospice program and resume active cancer treatment. You may go back into hospice care at a later time if needed. The hope is that hospice will improve your quality of life, making the best of each day during the last stages of advanced illness.

Hospice care services include the following:

- *Interdisciplinary team.* In most cases, an interdisciplinary team of doctors, nurses, pharmacists, social workers, home health aides, clergy, therapists, and trained volunteers provide care and offer support based on their areas of expertise.

- *Pain and symptom management.* The goal of pain and symptom control is to help you achieve comfort while allowing you to stay in control of your life. This means side effects are managed to make sure you are as pain and symptom free, and yet still as alert, as possible.

- *Spiritual care.* Your spiritual needs, as well as those of your family, are addressed. People differ in their spiritual and religious beliefs, so care is set up to meet the specific needs of your family. This service may help you explore what death means to you, say good-bye, or carry out certain religious ceremonies or rituals.

- *Home care and inpatient care.* Although hospice care is usually centered in the home, you may need to be admitted to the hospital, an extended-care facility, or an inpatient hospice facility. The hospice team can arrange and stay involved in your treatment and continue working with your family. You may resume in-home care when appropriate for you.

- *Respite care.* Your family and caregivers may at some point need time away from intense caregiving. Some hospice services may offer them a break through respite care, which is often done in 5-day periods. During this time, you will be cared for in either a hospice facility or in contracted beds in nursing homes or hospitals. Families can plan a mini-vacation, attend special events, or simply get some much-needed rest at home while you are cared for in an inpatient setting.

- *Family education.* Regularly scheduled meetings or conferences led by a member of the hospice team will keep your family members and caregivers informed of your condition and what to expect. These meetings also allow everyone to share their feelings, talk about expectations, and learn about death and the process of dying.

- *Bereavement care.* Bereavement is the time of mourning after a loss. The hospice care team works with surviving family and caregivers to help them through the grieving process. A trained volunteer, clergy member, or professional counselor provides support for the survivors through visits, phone calls, or letters, as well as through support groups. The team can make referrals for family members to other medical or professional care if needed. This service is usually provided to the family for about a year after a patient's death.

CHAPTER 10

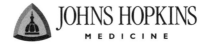

BRAIN CANCER IN OLDER ADULTS

BY GARY R. SHAPIRO, MD

Although the average age of the typical brain cancer patient is 55 years old, just over one-third of these tumors are now found in those older than 65 years. As we live longer, the number of men and women with cancers of the brain will increase dramatically. Since the 1970s, there has already been a seven-fold increase in the incidence of brain cancer in those older than 70 years, with the largest increases occurring in those older than 80 years of age.

Older adults with cancer often have other chronic health problems and may be taking multiple medications that can affect their cancer treatment plan. Prejudice, misunderstanding, and limited access to clinical trials often prevent older patients from getting the timely cancer treatment they need.

Intellectual decline, gait disturbance, short-term memory loss, and other symptoms of brain cancer may be mistaken-ly attributed to normal aging or dementia in seniors. When a cancer is found, it is too often ignored or undertreated. As a result, older individuals often have worse outcomes than younger patients.

WHY IS THERE MORE CANCER IN OLDER PEOPLE?

The organs in our body are made up of cells. Cells divide and multiply as the body needs them. Cancer develops when cells in a part of the body grow out of control. The body has a number of ways of repairing damaged control mechanisms, but as we get older, these do not work as well. Although our healthier lifestyles have allowed us to avoid death from infection, heart attack, and stroke, we may now live long enough for a cancer to develop. People who live longer have increased exposure to cancer-causing agents, or carcinogens, in the environment. Aging decreases the body's ability to protect us from these carcinogens and to repair cells that are damaged by these and other processes.

BRAIN CANCER IS DIFFERENT IN OLDER PEOPLE

Malignant gliomas, particularly glioblastoma multiforme, are the most common primary brain tumors in the elderly. Gliomas that appear before age 10 years and after age 45 years tend to be more aggressive and resistant to treatment than those that occur in other age groups. In seniors, even low-grade tumors are more aggressive than those seen in younger patients. Molecular biology studies indicate that there are specific age-related genetic alterations that deter-mine both the clinical course and response of brain tumors to therapy. Advanced age itself may be a risk factor for de-veloping brain cancer.

DECISION MAKING: 7 PRACTICAL STEPS

1. GET A DIAGNOSIS

No matter how "typical" the signs and symptoms, first impressions are sometimes wrong. A diagnosis helps you and your family understand what to expect and how to prepare for the future, even if you cannot get curative treatment. Knowing the diagnosis also helps your doctor treat your symptoms better. Many people find not knowing very hard and are relieved when they finally have an explanation for their symptoms. Sometimes, however, a frail patient is obviously dying, and diagnostic studies can be an additional burden. In such cases, it may be quite reasonable to focus on symptom relief, or palliation, without knowing the details of the diagnosis.

2. KNOW THE CANCER'S STAGE

There is no formal staging system for adult brain tumors. Instead, once a brain tumor has been diagnosed, the pathologist will perform several tests (see Chapter 1) on a tissue sample of the tumor to learn as much as possible about the tumor. Although factors like the location of the tumor in the brain and how much it has affected your neurologic function may be important, the cancer's tissue type (histology) and grade define your prognosis and treatment options. No one can make informed decisions without this information.

As it is in younger patients, histology and grade can only be determined by a biopsy. If resection is not possible, or the risks of surgery are too great, tissue from the brain tumor may be obtained by a stereotactic biopsy. As discussed in Step 1, the burdens of obtaining this tissue may be too great in a very frail, dying patient.

3. KNOW YOUR LIFE EXPECTANCY

Anticancer treatment should be considered if you are likely to live long enough to experience symptoms or premature death from brain cancer. If your life expectancy is so short that the cancer will not significantly affect it, there may be no reason to treat your cancer.

However, chronological age should not be the only thing that decides how your cancer should, or should not, be treated. Despite advanced age, people who are relatively well often have a life expectancy that is longer than their life expectancy with brain cancer. The average 70-year-old woman is likely to live another 16 years, and the average 70-year-old man another 12 years. A similar 85-year-old can expect to live an additional 5 to 6 years, and remain independent for most of that time. Even an unhealthy 75-year-old man or woman probably will live 5 to 6 more years— long enough to suffer symptoms and early death from recurrent brain cancer.

4. UNDERSTAND THE GOALS

The Goals of Treatment

It is important to be clear whether the goal of treatment is cure or palliation. If the goal is palliation, you need to understand if the treatment plan will extend your life, control your symptoms, or both. How likely is it to achieve these goals, and how long will you enjoy its benefits? More often than not, the goals of therapy are to control the tumor growth and to improve the patient's neurologic status.

When the goal of treatment is palliation, chemotherapy should never be administered without defined endpoints and timelines. It should be clear to everyone what "counts" as success, how it will be determined (for example, a symptom controlled or a smaller mass on CAT scan), and when. You and your family should understand what your options are at each step and how likely each option is to meet your goals. If this plan is not clear, ask your doctor to explain it in words you understand.

The Goals of the Patient

In addition to the traditional goals of tumor response, increased survival, and symptom control, older cancer patients often have goals related to quality of life. These goals may include maintaining physical and intellectual independence, spending quality time with family, taking trips, staying out of the hospital, or even sustaining economic stability. At times, palliative care or hospice may meet these goals better than active anticancer treatment. In addition to the medical team, older patients often turn to family, friends, and clergy to help guide them.

5. DETERMINE IF YOU ARE FIT OR FRAIL

Deciding how to treat cancer in someone who is older requires a thorough understanding of the individual's general health and social situation. Decisions about cancer treatment should never focus on age alone.

Age Is Not a Number

Your actual age has limited influence on how cancer will respond to therapy or its prognosis. Biologic changes and other changes associated with aging are more reliable in estimating an individual's vigor, life expectancy, or the risk of treatment complications. These changes include malnutrition, loss of muscle mass and strength, depression, dementia, falls, social isolation, and the inability to accomplish daily activities such as dressing, bathing, eating, shopping, housekeeping, and managing one's finances or medication.

Chronic Illnesses

Older cancer patients are likely to have chronic illnesses (comorbidities) that affect their life expectancy; the more a patient has, the greater the effect. This effect has little impact on the behavior of the cancer itself, but studies do show that comorbidities have a major impact on treatment outcome and its side effects.

6. BALANCE BENEFITS AND HARMS

Fit older brain cancer patients respond to treatment similarly to their younger counterparts. However, a word of caution is in order. Until recently, few studies included older individuals, and it may not be appropriate to apply these findings to the diverse group of older cancer patients.

The side effects of cancer treatment are never less in the elderly. In addition to the standard side effects, there are significant age-related toxicities to consider. Though most of these are more a function of frailty than chronological age, even the fittest senior cannot avoid the physical effects of aging. In addition to the changes in fat and muscle that a person sees in the mirror, there are age-related changes in kidney, liver, and digestive (gastrointestinal) functioning. These changes affect how the body absorbs and metabolizes anticancer drugs and other medicines. The average senior takes many different medicines (to control, for example, high blood pressure, high cholesterol, osteoporosis, diabetes, arthritis, etc.). This polypharmacy can cause undesirable side effects, as the many drugs interact with each other and the anticancer medications.

7. GET INVOLVED

Healthcare providers and family members often underestimate the physical and mental abilities of older people and their willingness to face chronic and life-threatening conditions. Studies clearly show that older patients want detailed and easily understood information about potential treatments and alternatives. Patients and families may consider cancer untreatable in the aged and may not understand the possibilities offered by treatment.

While patients with dementia pose a unique challenge, they are frequently capable of participating in goal setting and simple discussions about treatment side effects and logistics. Caring family members and friends are often able to share the patient's life story so that healthcare workers can work with them to make decisions consistent with the patient's values and desires. This communication of course is no substitute for a well–considered and properly executed living will or healthcare proxy.

While it is hard to face the possibility of life-threatening events at any age, it is always better to be prepared and to put your affairs in order. In addition to estate planning and wills, it is critical that you outline your wishes regarding medical care at the end of life and make legal provisions for someone to make those decisions if you are unable to make them for yourself.

TREATING BRAIN CANCER

YOU NEED A TEAM

Cancer care changes rapidly, and it is hard for the generalist to keep up to date, so referral to a specialist is essential. The needs of an older cancer patient often extend beyond the doctor's office and the traditional services provided by visiting nurses. These needs may include transportation, nutritional management, and emotional, financial, physical, or spiritual support. When an older individual with brain cancer is the primary caregiver for a frail or ill spouse, grandchildren, or other family members, special attention is necessary to provide for their needs as well. Older cancer patients cared for in geriatric oncology programs benefit from multidisciplinary teams of oncologists, geriatricians, psychiatrists, pharmacists, physiatrists, social workers, nurses, clergy, and dieticians, all working together as a team to identify and manage the stressors that can limit effective cancer treatment.

OVERVIEW

Except for some low-grade tumors, the treatments used for brain cancers are usually palliative. As discussed earlier, treatment decisions should be based not only on age, but also on life expectancy, performance status, and comorbid chronic illnesses. More aggressive therapy can benefit patients with good performance status and relatively small tumors that can be resected, especially those with favorable histologies and lower grades. For patients with debilitating medical problems, poor performance status, or significant neurologic deficit, it is reasonable to limit management to supportive care with corticosteroids, possibly including palliative radiation therapy.

Brain tumors are debilitating diseases that affect both cognitive and physical abilities. Physical and occupational therapy improve the patient's quality of life and ability to perform activities of daily living, even in those with a relatively short-term survival. Depression is a common problem in people who have brain tumors. It is usually more severe in older brain tumor patients and often requires treatment with antidepressant medicines. Care should be taken in choosing an appropriate antidepressant (SSRIs [selective serotonin reuptake inhibitors] are often preferred) since many of these agents, tricyclics and MAOIs (monoamine oxidase inhibitors), aggravate a number of medical problems that are common in older individuals: urinary retention related to an enlarged prostate, constipation, blurred vision, low blood pressure, rapid heart rate, and cognitive impairment. These same classes of antidepressants should not be taken with Matulane (procarbazine), a chemotherapeutic agent that is used to treat brain tumors.

SURGERY

Though brain cancer surgery is often complex, it is the standard of care for many cancers of the brain (see Chapter 3), regardless of age. Like other treatment options, surgery in some older individuals may involve risks related to decreases in body organ function (especially heart and lung), and it is essential that the surgeon and anesthetist work closely with your primary care physician (or a consultant) to fully assess and treat these problems before, during, and after the operation.

As in younger patients, survival rates depend on the histology, the grade, the location of the tumor in the brain, and the amount of tumor removed. Even when the entire tumor cannot be removed, debulking surgery does significantly increase survival, improve quality of life and performance status, and better the odds of response to subsequent radiation and chemotherapy. Brain surgery does have significantly higher risk in the elderly, especially those who have a poor performance status and other medical problems. Therefore, it is essential that you weigh all of the risks and benefits with your multidisciplinary care team.

RADIATION THERAPY

Radiation therapy (see Chapter 3) is often the treatment of choice for malignant brain tumors that occur in older individuals. It frequently improves both quality of life and survival. The fatigue that usually accompanies radiation therapy can be quite profound in the elderly, even in those who are fit. Often the logistical details (like daily travel to the hospital for a 6- to 7-week course of treatment) are the hardest for older people. It is important that you discuss these potential problems with your family and social worker prior to starting radiation therapy.

Accelerated fraction (hyperfractionation) radiation schedules (two or three daily treatments as opposed to one) have been used to deliver conventional doses of radiation over a shorter period of time. It is not the standard approach, and it is considered investigational by many radiation oncologists. Nevertheless, it may be something to consider in older individuals unable to tolerate the standard 6 to 7 weeks of daily radiation therapy. It is particularly suitable for those requiring hospitalization during treatment. Older individuals with a poor performance status may also want to consider hypofractionation radiation techniques. This investigational technique involves getting one fraction of radiation a week for about 6 weeks. Studies have shown improvements in survival and performance status in older patients when radiosensitizing doses of chemotherapy are also given.

Although the fatigue caused by radiation therapy usually resolves in a month or so, memory loss (usually short-term memory) and cognitive impairment are side effects that often do not improve. Although not widely accepted as an alternative to first-line palliative external beam radiation therapy (the type of radiation therapy used in the techniques discussed previously), stereotactic radiosurgery is an outpatient technique that allows the delivery of a single palliative fraction of high-dose radiation to a small, well-circumscribed tumor. It does not appear to cause any cognitive impairment.

CHEMOTHERAPY

Adding chemotherapy to radiation therapy does appear to prolong survival in many brain tumor patients. However, there have been few clinical trials focusing on the use of chemotherapy in older individuals. Nonfrail older cancer patients respond to chemotherapy (see Chapter 3) similarly to their younger counterparts. Reducing the dose of chemotherapy (or radiation therapy) based purely on chronological age may seriously affect the effectiveness of treatment. Managing chemotherapy-associated toxicity with appropriate supportive care is crucial in the elderly population to give them the best chance of cure and survival, or to provide the best palliation.

Though the side effects of cancer treatment are never less burdensome in the elderly, they can be managed by oncologists, especially geriatric oncologists, who work in teams with others who specialize in the care of the elderly. With appropriate care, healthy older patients do just as well with chemotherapy as younger patients. Advances in supportive care (antinausea medicines and blood cell growth factors) have significantly decreased the side effects of chemotherapy and improved safety and the quality of life of individuals with brain cancer. Nonetheless, there is risk, especially if the patient is frail. The presence of severe comorbidities, age-related frailty, or underlying severe psychosocial problems may be obstacles for highly intensive treatment plans. Such patients may benefit from less complicated or potentially less toxic treatment plans.

COMMON TREATMENT COMPLICATIONS IN THE ELDERLY

Corticosteroids (Decadron, prednisone) are used in patients with brain tumors to decrease the brain swelling (edema) caused by the tumor and its treatment. It is not unusual for a patient with symptoms of brain edema (confusion, lethargy, neurologic deficit) to show a dramatic improvement shortly after beginning this medication. Corticosteroids do have a number of side effects that can be particularly problematic, and are not at all uncommon in older individuals, especially those who already have these problems: gastric irritation, depression, psychosis, fluid retention (triggering congestive heart failure), and elevated blood sugar (diabetes). Muscle weakness, or myopathy, and osteoporosis can also be a problem in those who live long enough. There is often no choice but to use corticosteroids in brain tumor patients, and it is essential that older individuals are carefully monitored and that their doctors use appropriate precautionary measures, such as the liberal use of antacids. Sometimes diuretics can be used to decrease brain edema in individuals with specific high-risk contraindications to corticosteroids, such as active peptic ulcer disease, serious congestive heart failure, or uncontrolled diabetes.

Anemia (low red blood cell count) is common in the elderly, especially those that are frail. It decreases the effectiveness of chemotherapy and often causes fatigue, falls, cognitive decline (e.g., dementia, disorientation, confusion), and heart problems. Therefore, it is essential that anemia be recognized and corrected with red blood cell transfusions or the appropriate use of erythropoiesis-stimulating agents like Procrit, Epogen, or Aranesp.

Myelosuppression (low white blood cell count) is also common in older patients receiving chemotherapy or radiation therapy. Older patients with myelosuppression develop life-threatening infections more often than younger patients, and they may need to be treated in the hospital for many days. The liberal use of granulopoietic growth factors (Neupogen [filgrastim], Neulasta [pegfilgrastim]) decreases the risk of infection and makes it possible for older individuals to receive full doses of chemotherapy.

Mucositis (mouth sores) and diarrhea can cause severe dehydration in older patients, who often are already dehydrated due to inadequate fluid intake and diuretics (water pills taken for high blood pressure or heart failure). Careful monitoring and the liberal use of antidiarrheal agents such as Imodium (loperamide) as well as oral and intravenous fluids are essential components of the management of older cancer patients.

Kidney function declines as we age. Some of the medicines that older patients take to treat both their cancer (e.g., Platinol AQ [cisplatin], Paraplatin [carboplatin], nonsteroidal anti-inflammatory drugs) and non-cancer-related problems might further worsen kidney function. The dehydration that often accompanies cancer and its treatment can put additional stress on the kidneys. Fortunately, it is often possible to minimize these effects by carefully selecting and dosing appropriate drugs, managing polypharmacy, and preventing dehydration.

Neurotoxicity and cognitive effects, or chemo brain, can be profoundly debilitating in patients who are already cognitively impaired (e.g., demented, disoriented, confused). As discussed previously, radiation therapy and brain surgery often impair cognition. Elderly patients with a history of falling, hearing loss, or peripheral neuropathy (nerve damage from, for example, diabetes) have decreased energy and are highly vulnerable to neurotoxic chemotherapy such as the taxanes or platinum compounds. Many of the medicines used to control nausea (antiemetics) or decrease the side effects of certain chemotherapeutic agents are also potential neurotoxins. These medicines include Decadron, which can cause psychosis and agitation; Zantac (ranitidine), which can cause agitation; and Benadryl (diphenhydramine) and some of the antiemetics, which can cause sedation.

Fatigue is a near-universal complaint of older cancer patients. Radiation therapy will probably make it worse. It is particularly a problem for those who are socially isolated or depend upon others to help them with activities of daily living. It is not necessarily related to depression, but it can be. Depression is quite common in the elderly. In contrast to younger patients who often respond to a cancer diagnosis with anxiety, depression is the more common disorder in older cancer patients. With proper support and medical attention (see Chapter 4), many of these patients can safely receive anticancer treatment.

Heart problems increase with age, and it is no surprise that older cancer patients have an increased risk of cardiac complications from intensive surgery, radiation, and chemotherapy. Patients treated with cisplatin chemotherapy require large amounts of intravenous fluid hydration. This can cause congestive heart failure in patients with heart problems; they need careful monitoring (as do those receiving corticosteroids—discussed earlier in this section). Atherosclerosis (blood vessel damage from hardening of the arteries) may increase the chances of local radiation therapy toxicity. Lung problems (especially pulmonary fibrosis) may occur in those receiving BCNU, especially those who have underlying chronic obstructive pulmonary disease or emphysema.

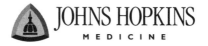

CHAPTER 11

TRUSTED RESOURCES—FINDING ADDITIONAL INFORMATION ABOUT BRAIN CANCER AND ITS TREATMENT

F or those of you wanting more information about brain cancer, there is a large amount of educational materials and resources, both financial and emotional, available from many organizations. The following is a list of trusted and useful Web sites and organizations that may be able to further assist you.

BRAIN TUMOR WEB SITES

Adult Brain Tumor Consortium (ABTC)
http://www.abtconsortium.org

The ABTC is a multi-institutional consortium created from the consolidation of the New Approaches to Brain Tumor

Therapy (NABTT) and the North American Brain Tumor Consortium (NABTC), which were both funded by the NCI. ABTC allows investigators from NABTT and NABTC to continue their research while centralizing the management of their programs into a single entity.

American Brain Tumor Association (ABTA)

http://www.abta.org
(800) 886-2282

The ABTA is a nonprofit organization whose goal is promoting research on brain tumors and also offers support and information to patients affected by brain tumors and their loved ones.

The Healing Exchange Brain Trust

http://www.braintrust.org
(877) 252-8480

The Healing Exchange Brain Trust runs a number of online support groups, including the BRAINTMR list, which is a forum for topics related to all types of brain tumors. Information and experience is shared here among patients and their loved ones, researchers, health professionals, and educators.

International Brain Tumour Alliance (IBTA)

http://www.theibta.org

The IBTA provides support, advocacy, and information to brain tumor patients, researchers, scientists, and healthcare professionals to countries all over the world.

Musella Foundation for Brain Tumor Research and Information/Virtual Trials

http://www.virtualtrials.com/musella.cfm
(888) 295-4740

The Musella Foundation works to improve the lives and survival rates of patients with brain tumors by organizing the brain tumor community, streamlining the flow of information, and raising money for research using technology. The Musella Foundation also maintains "Virtual Trials," which allows patients to document their specific treatment history. Treatment combinations that provided longer survivals or better quality of life for patients are then evaluated to identify potential new promising treatment regimens.

National Brain Tumor Society (NBTS)

http://www.braintumor.org
(800) 770-8287
(800) 934-CURE (2873)

The NBTS brings together the best of patient services and research to be a comprehensive resource for patients and their loved ones, researchers, and medical professionals. A leader in the brain tumor community, NBTS was formed after the Brain Tumor Society and the National Brain Tumor Foundation merged in 2008. These organizations were formed by parents and other concerned individuals who were committed to increasing funding for research and patient access to brain tumor resources.

CANCER AND CLINICAL TRIAL-RELATED WEB SITES

American Cancer Society

http://www.cancer.org

(800) ACS-2345 (227-2345)

The American Cancer Society is a nationwide voluntary health organization dedicated to eliminating cancer and learning more about its prevention, treatment, and symptom relief through advocacy, research, education, and service.

American Society of Clinical Oncology (ASCO)

http://www.asco.org

(888) 282-2552

Founded in 1964, ASCO is a nonprofit organization whose members include over 27,000 healthcare professionals from all oncology disciplines who are working to improve cancer care and prevention.

Cancer Hope Network

http://www.cancerhopenetwork.org

(800) 552-4366

Cancer Hope Network provides confidential and free individual support for cancer patients and their loved ones.

Cancer*Care*, Inc.

http://www.cancercare.org

(800) 813-HOPE (4673)

Cancer*Care* provides free support services to anyone affected by cancer, including patients, their loved ones, and caregivers. Support services are provided by oncology social workers and include education, financial assistance, counseling and support groups, and practical help.

CenterWatch

http://www.centerwatch.com

(866) 219-3440

This service provides comprehensive details regarding clinical trials.

Coalition of Cancer Cooperative Groups

http://www.cancertrialshelp.org

(877) 520-4457

The mission of the Coalition of Cancer Cooperative Groups is to improve patient awareness of, access to, and participation in cancer clinical trials. The Coalition identifies cancer research issues and works to overcome them.

CURE: Cancer Updates, Research & Education

http://www.curetoday.com

(800) 210-CURE (2873)

CURE Media Group publishes CURE magazine as a guide for the cancer experience. The recipient of a national nursing award, CURE uses this magazine, books, online tools, educational forums, and a resource guide for the newly diagnosed to try to make cancer understandable for patients.

National Cancer Institute

http://www.cancer.gov

(800) 4-CANCER (422-6237)

Established under the National Cancer Institute Act of 1937, the NCI is the premier agency for cancer research and cancer care training. The NCI's National Cancer Program supports and conducts training; research; health information dissemination; and programs that investigate the prevention, diagnosis, cause, treatment of, and rehabilitation from cancer; as well as continued care for patients and patients' loved ones.

National Coalition for Cancer Survivorship (NCCS)
http://www.canceradvocacy.org
(888) 650-9127

The NCCS is a cancer advocacy organization that advocates for changes in how the nation finances, researches, regulates, and delivers quality cancer care. NCCS runs Cancer Advocacy Now!, a legislative network that engages representatives in cancer-related issues on the federal level, and also produces the Cancer Survival Toolbox for cancer patients.

FINANCIAL ASSISTANCE/ADVOCACY

Cancer Fund of America
http://www.cfoa.org

Cancer Fund of America helps cancer patients, hospices, and other nonprofit healthcare providers by directly sending them free products.

Hill-Burton Free Health Care
http://www.hrsa.gov/gethealthcare/affordable/
hillburton/
(800) 638-0742

Congress passed a law in 1946 giving healthcare facilities loans and grants for modernization and construction in exchange for their providing some services to those unable to pay for them, as well as to those who live in the area of the facility. Funding was stopped in 1997, but there are still about 200 facilities that provide care that is free or reduced in cost.

National Association for the Terminally Ill (NATI)
http://www.healthfinder.gov/orgs/HR3440.htm
(866) 668-1724

NATI offers financial help to the families of terminally ill patients with a life expectancy of less than two years in order to help them again be financially independent. NATI offers two programs that do this, the Life-Threatening Illness Program and Children and Family Cancer Program. NATI also helps the needy and elderly in getting medicines and medical equipment.

Patient Advocate Foundation (PAF)
http://www.patientadvocate.org
http://www.copays.org
(800) 532-5274

PAF provides mediation and arbitration services to help chronically and terminally ill patients with insurance and employment issues and medical debt crises.

Social Security Administration
http://www.ssa.gov
(800) 772-1213

The Social Security Administration is the official US government agency responsible for disability for the chronically ill as well as survivor benefits.

MEDICATION ASSISTANCE

Each state in the United States has an agency whose purpose is to provide assistance in receiving medical care and treatment for its residents providing they meet eligibility criteria. See your individual states' homepage for access.

Needy Meds
http://www.needymeds.com

NeedyMeds helps people who struggle to afford health care and medicine. These services are free and information is offered anonymously.

Partnership for Prescription Assistance (PPA)
http://www.pparx.org
(888) 4PPA-NOW (477-2669)

PPA offers programs to help patients without prescription drug coverage who qualify get their medicines. Many will get their medications free or nearly free.

RxAssist
http://www.rxassist.org
(401) 729-3284

RxAssist provides access to a database of pharmaceutical company-run patient assistance programs that provide free medications to people in need. RxAssist also offers news, articles, and practical tools to patients and healthcare professionals.

SUPPORT AND ASSISTANCE

Hospice Education Institute
http://www.hospiceworld.org
(800) 331-1620

The Hospice Education Institute offers education and information about caring for the bereaved and the dying to the public and healthcare professionals.

National Association of Hospital Hospitality Houses (NAHHH)
http://www.nahhh.org
(800) 542-9730

The NAHHH supports hospital hospitality homes to be more effective in their services and provides resources for patients and families.

National Family Caregivers Association (NFCA)
http://www.nfcacares.org
(800) 896-3650

The NFCA provides education, support, and advocacy to family caregivers of the chronically ill, disabled, or elderly in the United States.

National Hospice and Palliative Care Organization (NHPCO)
http://nhpco.org
(800) 658-8898

NHPCO represents palliative care and hospice programs and professionals throughout the US and works to increase access to and improve end-of-life care.

National Students of Ailing Mothers and Fathers (AMF)
Support Network
http://www.studentsofamf.org

This organization offers support for college students who have a parent with cancer or who have lost a parent to cancer.

TRANSPORTATION ASSISTANCE
Air Care Alliance
http://www.aircareall.org
(888) 260-9707

The Air Care Alliance is a league of humanitarian flying organizations in the United States whose pilots are dedicated to community service. Their Web site provides an overview of all these organizations that perform public benefit flying for patient transport, health care, disaster relief, and more.

Corporate Angel Network

http://www.corpangelnetwork.org

(866) 328-1313

The Corporate Angel Network sets up free flights to treatment centers for cancer patients to lessen the stress, discomfort, and cost of travel.

Mercy Medical Airlift

http://www.mercymedical.org

(800) 296-1217

Mercy Medical Airlift is an organization that is dedicated to helping those in need by providing free air medical transportation.

US Air Ambulance

http://www.usairambulance.com

(800) 971-4351

US Air Ambulance is a fee-for-service company that provides aero-medical transport nationally and internationally.

TREATMENT RESOURCES

CancerSource.com

http://www.angelsofhope.net/cancersource.html

(770) 631-6761

CancerSource.com offers free services and information to cancer patients and their caregivers by providing personalized access to cancer resources.

Chemocare.com

http://www.chemocare.com

Chemocare.com was set up by cancer survivor Scott Hamilton to make accessible the latest chemotherapy information to patients and their families, friends, and caregivers as a supplement to the information provided by their healthcare providers.

Temodar.com

http://www.temodar.com

Temodar.com has PDFs that offer information on brain tumors and their treatment for patients and caregivers. Information about brain tumor types and symptoms, as well as management of side effects and coping tips, is given.

OTHER RELATED SITES

American Pain Foundation (APF)

http://www.painfoundation.org

(888) 615-PAIN (7246)

The American Pain Foundation provides support, information, and advocacy to those suffering from pain. They work for quality of life by increasing awareness, promoting research, and providing information to make effective pain management more accessible.

Brain Injury Association of America (BIAA)

http://www.biausa.org

(703) 761-0750

The BIAA offers education, information, and support for patients, their families, and the professionals who are affected by brain injuries. With a network of hundreds of local chapters and support groups and more than 40 chartered state affiliates, the BIAA works to promote awareness and provide more access to quality health care.

Caregiver.com

http://www.caregiver.com

(800) 829-2734

Caregiver Media Group is dedicated to providing guidance, information, and support for families and caregivers. They produce *Today's Caregiver*, which is a national magazine for caregivers; the "Fearless Caregiver Conferences"; and a Web site that includes chat rooms, online discussion lists, an online store, newsletters, and back issues of *Today's Caregiver*. Everything produced by Caregiver Media Group is made for, about, and by caregivers.

Disability Resources, Inc.
http://www.disabilityresources.org

Disability Resources, Inc. works to raise awareness and make available accessible information that can help people with disabilities.

Healthfinder
http://www.healthfinder.gov

Healthfinder.gov is a government-run Web site that offers tools, information, and tips to help you and your loved ones stay healthy.

National Aphasia Association (NAA)
http://www.aphasia.org
(800) 922-4622

The NAA promotes rehabilitation, education, research, and support services to people with aphasia and their loved ones.

National Center for Complementary and Alternative Medicine (NCCAM)
http://www.nccam.nih.gov
(888) 644-6226

The NCCAM is the government's lead agency for scientific research on the diverse medical and healthcare systems, practices, and products that are not generally considered part of conventional medicine and are known as complementary and alternative medicine.

Visiting Nurse Associations of America (VNAA)

http://www.vnaa.org
(202) 384-1420

The VNAA advocates for, supports, and promotes community-based home hospice and healthcare providers to care for all individuals.

Vital Options International

http://www.vitaloptions.org
(818) 508-5657

Vital Options works with the professional oncology and patient advocacy communities, allowing patients and their loved ones to interact directly with worldwide oncology opinion leaders about the latest advances in cancer advocacy, research, treatment, and public policy issues. All Vital Options services are free.

Well Spouse Foundation (WSA)

http://www.wellspouse.org

The Well Spouse Association advocates for the needs of caregivers for chronically ill and/or disabled spouses/partners. The WSA offers support for the caregivers and educates the public about the difficulties caregivers face every day.

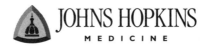

The Johns Hopkins Comprehensive Brain Tumor Center at Johns Hopkins

http://www.hopkinsmedicine.org/neurology_
neurosurgery/specialty_areas/brain_tumor/

The Johns Hopkins Comprehensive Brain Tumor Center in Baltimore, Maryland, is one of the largest brain tumor treatment and research centers in the world. They treat an extremely large number of patients affected by all types of brain tumors and tailor the best and most advanced therapies that each unique tumor demands.

Treatment for patients with brain tumors is best done by a multidisciplinary team that includes tumor physicians from various medical specialties, including but not limited to neurosurgeons, neuro-oncologists, radiation therapists, and pathologists. At the Johns Hopkins Comprehensive Brain Tumor Center, weekly mutlidisciplinary brain tumor conferences are held with all medical specialties present to review each tumor case and make the best diagnosis and treatment plan for the individual patient. The team consists of skilled surgeons and neurologists that can provide the most effective and safest treatment—even on the most challenging types of tumors.

In addition, the research program has an unparalleled history of introducing new forms of treatment for the patients affected by malignant brain tumors. A national leading role in the design and the completion of multi-center clinical trials allows Johns Hopkins to apply the most promising discoveries from the laboratory to patient care in an effective and expeditious fashion.

The strong team of experts at Johns Hopkins work closely together in a rigorous interdisciplinary fashion and combines the latest imaging and modern monitoring methods to offer an unparalleled variety of treatment approaches. In addition, the strong support staff assists patients and families coping with these difficult diagnoses.

About Johns Hopkins Medicine

Johns Hopkins Medicine unites physicians and scientists of the Johns Hopkins School of Medicine with the organizations, health professionals, and facilities of the Johns Hopkins Health System. Its mission is to improve the health of the community and the world by setting the standard of excellence in the medical education, research, and clinical care. Diverse and inclusive, Johns Hopkins Medicine has provided international leadership in the education of physicians and medical scientists in biomedical research and in the application of medical knowledge to sustain health since The Johns Hopkins Hospital opened in 1889.

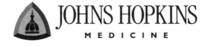

FURTHER READING

100 Questions & Answers About Brain Tumors, Second Edition, Virginia Stark-Vance, MD, and Mary Louise Dubay; Jones & Bartlett Learning, 2011.

100 Questions & Answers About Head and Brain Injuries, Rahul Jandial, MD; Jones & Bartlett Learning, 2009.

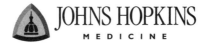

GLOSSARY

Adjuvant therapy: Treatment given after the primary treatment to increase the chances of a cure, and treatment to prevent the cancer from recurring.

Adrenocorticosteroid: A hormone that is normally made in the adrenal cortex or the kidney. Often synthetic adrenocorticosteriods are given to patients with brain tumors to help control or minimize cerebral edema and swelling. The most commonly used steroid is Decadron.

Advance directives: Legal documents, including living wills and durable power of attorney, that allow people to express their decisions regarding what they do and don't want to have done during their last weeks or months in case they become unable to communicate effectively.

Alopecia: Hair loss that can be complete or just a thinning of scalp hair.

Alternative therapy: Medicines used in lieu of standard medical therapies.

Anemia: A condition in which the number of red blood cells is less than normal.

Antiemetics: Antinausea medications.

Antiepileptic drugs (AEDs): AEDs belong to a diverse group of pharmaceuticals used in the treatment of seizures. The goal of an AED is to suppress the rapid and excessive firing of neurons that start a seizure. Effective AEDs would prevent the spread of the seizure within the brain. AEDs are also known as anticonvulsants and antiseizure drugs.

Baseline study: Usually MRIs that serve as a point of comparison used to determine if the tumor is responding to treatment. Ideally postoperative baseline studies should occur within 72 hours of surgery.

BCNU: Another name for the chemotherapeutic drug carmustine. BCNU is classified as an alkylating agent and its cytotoxic effects come from stopping cells from dividing and therefore cause cell death. BCNU is available in two forms: both a locally implantable impregnated dissolvable wafer and an intravenous form for systemic delivery.

Benign: Any tumor or growth that is not malignant or cancerous. A benign growth will not spread, or metastasize, to other areas of the body.

Biopsy: A procedure in which cells are collected for microscopic examination.

Blood clots: A blood clot, also known as a thrombus, is a clump that forms in the blood when the blood hardens from a liquid to a solid.

Brain: The brain is a soft, spongy mass of nerve cells and supportive tissue that is responsible for the generation of the signals that control the neurologic function of the body. It has six main divisions: the frontal, parietal, temporal, and occipital lobes; the brain stem; and the cerebellum. In the center of the brain are four connected hollow spaces called ventricles. The ventricles contain a clear water-like liquid called cerebrospinal fluid that circulates throughout the central nervous system.

Cancer: The presence of malignant cells.

Cancer survivor: Cancer survivors can be people who live with cancer, including those with terminal cancer, and can also be family members, friends, and caregivers of those who have been diagnosed with cancer.

Cancerous: A cell or mass is said to be cancerous when it is malignant, or growing rapidly and out of control.

Carcinogen: Cancer-causing substance.

Carcinomas: Cancers that form in the surface cells of different tissues.

Cells: Basic elements of tissues; the appearance and composition of individual cells are unique to the tissue they compose.

Central nervous system (CNS): The CNS is composed of the brain and spinal cord. This book focuses on malignant gliomas, which occur mainly in the brain but in very rare instances can spread to the spinal cord.

Cerebrospinal fluid (CSF): Cerebrospinal fluid is a clear liquid that surrounds the brain and spinal cord. It cushions and protects the brain against injury and circulates through the four ventricles and bathes the brain. The CNS has a closed circulatory fluid system that drains into the bloodstream.

Chemo brain: Difficulty with cognitive functioning as a side effect of receiving chemotherapy.

Chemotherapy: The use of chemical agents (drugs) to systemically treat cancer.

Clinical trial: A study of a drug or treatment with a large group of people testing the treatment.

Cognitive dysfunction: A difficulty with concentration, memory, arithmetic, or the ability to make appropriate decisions. This can be caused by damage or swelling in the brain or can be associated with systemic treatment and stress.

Comorbidity: A disease or disorder someone already has prior to a new diagnosis. Examples include diabetes, heart disease, and a previous history of blood clots.

Complementary therapy: Medicines used in conjunction with standard therapies.

Computed Tomography (CAT) scan: Computerized series of X-rays that create a detailed cross-sectional image of the body. CAT images can help identify some types of tumors, as well as help detect swelling, bleeding, and bone and tissue calcification.

Corticosteroids: This is a class of steroid hormones that is produced in the adrenal cortex. Brain tumor patients frequently require corticosteroid medications such as dexamethasone to help control swelling in the brain.

Craniotomy: An operation that removes a piece of skull to allow access to the brain.

Cytotoxic: The ability to kill fast-growing cells, both cancerous and noncancerous, by preventing them from dividing.

Drain: A small tube inserted into a wound cavity to collect fluid.

Durable power of attorney: A document that specifies a family member to have legal authority to make all decisions, personal and financial, for you in case you become incapacitated. The information in this document is usually based on prior discussions of wishes.

Edema: Swelling in the brain caused by fluid trapped in tissue/ brain tissue.

Epileptologist: A neurologist whose specialty is treating epilepsy or seizure disorders. Epileptologists are generally consulted when seizures fail to stop when first treated.

External beam radiotherapy: Delivers radiation waves more focally and reduces the likelihood of radiation spread to structures beyond the targeted tumor tissue within the brain.

Functional Magnetic Resonance Imaging (fMRI): This special MRI requires patients to speak, read, and follow commands during an MRI. These tasks require extra blood to be sent to the parts of the brain responsible for the specific function. fMRIs measure the blood flow and provide images outlining these "functional" areas. These images will assist your surgeon in planning and performing your resection by helping to guide the removal of non-eloquent tissue and preserve those areas of your brain that are functional.

Genetic mutation: A gene with a mistake or alteration.

Gliadel: This is an FDA-approved chemotherapeutic implant for use during neurosurgical resection of both newly diagnosed and recurrent high-grade malignant gliomas (WHO III & IV).

Glioma: A tumor that arises in the central nervous system. Gliomas are most commonly found in the brain, and are the most common brain tumor. They are graded or classified by the World Health Organization (WHO) from I–IV (1–4), grade I being the most indolent or benign and grade IV being the most aggressive or malignant.

Grade: The grade of a cancer describes the cancer's level of aggression.

Guided imagery: A mind–body technique in which the patient visualizes and meditates on images that encourage a positive immune response.

Healthcare proxy: A document that permits a designated person to make decisions regarding your medical treatment when you are unable to do so.

Histologic tumor grade: Describes the speed of the cancer's growth and its level of aggression.

Hospice: Approaches and support to help with end-of-life care, including personal care, symptom control, and quality of life. End-of-life care may occur at home or in an inpatient hospice setting. Hospice providers can also help with bereavement issues for the patient and family.

Immunotherapy: The use of immune cells to treat cancer.

Incidence: The number of times a disease occurs within a population of people.

Infiltrative: There are no clear borders between the cancerous area and the surrounding brain.

Informed consent: A process that includes the healthcare provider or physician describing in detail the proposed procedure or treatment as well as all of the risks and benefits associated with it. The patient or his or her legal guardian, the physician, and a witness must sign a form describing the details of the discussion, which gives permission to proceed. This is a legal document.

Initial therapy: Treatment given as the first approach. In brain cancer, initial therapy is often surgery.

Interstitial brachytherapy: Treatment that includes placing radioactive materials within a tumor cavity.

Intraoperative frozen section: An examination of a tumor sample by a pathologist during a surgical procedure that provides preliminary information about what type of tumor the patient has. This reading may be changed once the final permanent pathology slides are made.

Invasive cancer: Cancer that grows and invades into areas surrounding the initial site where the cancer started.

Living will: A document that outlines what care you want in the event that you become unable to communicate due to coma or heavy sedation.

Local therapy: A treatment, in the form of chemotherapy or radiation, that is placed directly into the cavity where the tumor was removed.

Lymphatic system: A collection of vessels with the principal functions of transporting digested fat from the intestine to the bloodstream, removing and destroying toxins from tissues, and resisting the spread of disease throughout the body.

Magnetic Resonance Imaging (MRI): A scanning device that uses magnetic fields and computers to capture images of the brain on screen and on film. It provides pictures from various planes, or visual "slices" of the brain, that can be combined on-screen to create a three-dimensional image of the tumor. The MRI detects signals emitted from normal and abnormal tissue, providing detailed views of the brain anatomy and any areas of abnormality.

Malignant: Cancerous; growing rapidly and out of control.

Median survival: Also called median overall survival, this is the time from diagnosis or treatment at which half of the patients with a given disease are expected or found to still be alive. In a clinical trial, median survival time is use to measure how effective a treatment is.

Meninges: Layers of tissue that act as protective membranes and surround the brain and spinal cord. The dura mater, which is the outermost layer, is thick and leather-like, while the second and third layers (the arachnoid and the pia mater) are thin.

Metastasis, metastasize: The spread of cancer to other organ sites.

Mortality: The statistical calculation of death rates due to a specific disease within a population.

Mucositis: Inflammation and sores in the mouth and throat that usually arise from systemic therapy.

Mutated: Altered.

Myelosuppression: Low white blood cell count.

National Cancer Institute (NCI): Established under the National Cancer Institute Act of 1937, the NCI is the premier agency for cancer research and cancer care training. The NCI's National Cancer Program supports and conducts training; research; health information dissemination; and programs that investigate the prevention, diagnosis, cause, treatment of, and rehabilitation from cancer; as well as continued care for patients and patients' loved ones.

National Comprehensive Cancer Network (NCCN): The NCCN is an alliance of leading cancer centers whose goal is to improve both the effectiveness and the quality of the care that patients receive. NCCN works to achieve this by developing resources and clinical practice guidelines for patients, clinicians, and others in health care.

Neurosurgeon/Neurosurgical oncologist: A specialist trained in the surgical removal of cancerous tumors from the brain.

Neurotoxicity: Adverse effects on the structure or function of the central and/or peripheral nervous system caused by exposure to a toxic chemical.

Neutropenia: A decrease in the number of neutrophils, or white blood cells, in the blood. White blood cells are the cells in the blood that help fight infection.

Nonsteroidal anti-inflammatory drug (NSAID): A class of pain medications, often sold over the counter, that includes Advil and similar common pain killers.

Oncologist/Neuro-oncologist: A cancer specialist trained to determine treatment choices and treat cancer, primarily with drugs or medications. Those who have specialized training and treat only patients with cancer of the brain and central nervous system are neuro-oncologists.

Oncology nurses: Specially trained nurses that provide care and support for patients diagnosed with cancer. They are responsible for administering chemotherapy and managing symptoms related to cancer illnesses.

Open procedures: Surgical procedures in which an incision is made to visualize the organs and tissue to be removed.

Opioids: Medicines derived from morphine and similar chemicals and used to treat pain.

Palliative care: Care to relieve the symptoms of cancer and to keep the best quality of life for as long as possible when cure is no longer the goal.

Paralysis: Paralysis is the loss of function in one or more muscles that can be accompanied by a lack of feeling in that area due to sensory damage.

Paresis: A condition typified by partial loss of movement or impaired movement.

Pathologist/Neuropathologist: A specialist trained to distinguish normal from abnormal cells. Those who have specialized training in identifying cancer of the brain and central nervous system are neuropathologists.

Peripheral neuropathy: Tingling, numbness, or burning sensation in hands, feet, or legs caused by damage to peripheral nerves by a tumor or by chemotherapy or radiation.

Phases: A series of steps followed in clinical trials to test and develop a new drug or combination of drugs. Phase I aims to define the tolerated dose, safety, and toxicity of a new drug or new combination of drugs. Phase II aims to define how effective a new drug or combination is in treating a specific disease and to further define safety and toxicity. Phase III aims to define how effective a new drug or combination is when compared with the current standard treatment for a specific disease.

Placebos: An inert treatment, such as sugar pills, given in some clinical trials to determine how much of a medicine's value is psychological.

Platelets: Small blood cells that prevent bleeding by forming clots at sites of injury.

Post traumatic stress disorder (PTSD): Emotional disorder resulting in a high level of anxiety and sometimes depression caused by a traumatic event in the past.

Preoperative tests: Tests done to ensure that there are no acute health conditions requiring attention prior to undergoing surgery or radiation.

Primary care doctor: Regular physician who gives medical check-ups and treatment of noncancer-related illness.

Primary or intrinsic: Primary or intrinsic brain tumors originate in the brain and rarely spread to anywhere outside of the CNS.

Primary treatment/therapy: The initial cancer treatment. Primary treatment for brain cancer usually involves surgery for resection or biopsy.

Prognosis: An estimation of the likely outcome of an illness based upon the patient's current status and the available treatments.

Protocol: The treatment plan that can be research or standard accepted treatment and provides information about how, when, and to whom a drug or treatment is given.

Psychosocial support staff: Staff who assist in coping with stress associated with diagnosis through recovery and beyond.

Pulmonary embolism (PE): A blood clot that forms somewhere in the body, usually in the lower legs, and circulates to the lungs, causing full or partial blockage of one or both pulmonary arteries.

Radiation oncologist: A physician specializing in the treatment of disease using radiation therapy. The radiation oncologist works with the radiation physicist to determine the amount of radiation therapy required and oversees the delivery of radiation therapy treatment.

Radiation physicist: Works with radiation oncologists to determine the amount of radiation required for treatment. The radiation physicist also makes sure that the equipment is working properly and that the machines deliver the correct dose of radiation.

Radiation therapist: A person who positions the patients for radiation treatments and runs the equipment that delivers the radiation.

Radiation therapy: Use of high-energy X-rays to kill cancer cells and shrink tumors. Radiation therapy is often also referred to as "fractionated external beam radiation therapy," which simply means it is divided into smaller treatments delivered daily called fractions. The radiation is delivered from an external source hence the external beam.

Radiologist/Neuroradiologist: A specialist trained to read and interpret radiological tests such as X-rays, CAT scans, and MRIs to diagnose and treat a disease. Those who have specialized training in identifying abnormalities of the brain and CNS are neuroradiologists.

Recurrent cancer: A disease that has come back in spite of the initial treatment.

Red blood cells: Cells in the blood whose primary function is to carry oxygen to tissues.

Resection: The surgical removal, either in part or completely, of an organ or lesion.

Risk factors: Any factors that contribute to an increased possibility of getting cancer.

Seizure: A seizure results from abnormal activity in the brain. Seizures can present in several ways, ranging from thrashing movements, known as tonic-clonic seizures, to brief losses of consciousness.

Sexual dysfunction: Difficulty with sexual function that can encompass impotence (lack of erection), loss of lubrication, painful intercourse, or a loss of interest in sex that can result from cancer symptoms or treatment.

Side effects: Unintended symptoms produced by a therapy.

Skull: The framework of 8 cranial and 14 facial bones that protect the brain. The cranium, the part of the skull that covers the brain, is made up of four major bones: the frontal, occipital, sphenoid, and ethmoid bones. There are four other bones in the cranium: two temporal bones, which are located on the sides and base of the skull, and two parietal bones, which fuse at the top of the skull. The areas where the bones in the skull meet are called sutures.

Social worker: This professional is involved in support issues surrounding the management of brain cancer and also in addressing financial concerns.

Surgical biopsy: The removal of a portion of the tissue for further evaluation and diagnosis.

Surgical margin: Visible normal tissue removed with surgical excision of a tumor.

Survivor volunteer: This individual "who has been there before" can offer tremendous emotional support and complements the service the professional staff provides.

Systemic treatment: A treatment that affects the whole body, such as oral or intravenous treatment.

Targeted therapy: Treatment that targets specific molecules involved in carcinogenesis or tumor growth.

Thrombocytopenia: An abnormal drop in the number of blood cells involved in forming blood clots. These cells are called platelets.

Thrombosis: Another name for a blood clot.

Thrush: Fungal or yeast infection of the mucosa in the mouth.

Tumor: A mass or lump of tissue that is abnormal.

Ventricles: Four connected and fluid-filled cavities in the center of the brain that hold the CSF.

Ventriculoperitoneal shunt: A catheter surgically inserted into one of the lateral ventricles of the brain to drain CSF out of the brain via a tube tunneled under the skin. The CSF is drained into the abdominal cavity, and this is done when normal drainage pathways are not working.

World Health Organization (WHO): The WHO, established in 1948 and headquartered in Geneva, Switzerland, is a specialized branch of the United Nations that oversees international public health.

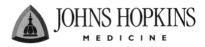